Created by Xspurts.com

All rights reserved.

Copyright © 2005 onwards .

By reading this book, you agree to the below Terms and Conditions.

Xspurts.com retains all rights to these products.

No part of this book may be reproduced in any form, by photostat, microfilm, xerography, or any other means, or incorporated into any information retrieval system, electronic or mechanical, without the written permission of Xspurts.com; exceptions are made for brief excerpts used in published reviews.

This publication is designed to provide accurate and authoritative information with regard to the subject matter covered but is for entertainment purposes only. It is sold with the understanding that the publisher is not engaged in rendering legal, accounting, health, relationship or other professional / personal advice. If legal advice or other expert assistance is required, the services of a competent professional should be sought.

♥ A New Zealand Designed Product

Get A Free Book At: https://free.xspurts.com

XSPURTS

Table of Contents:

Table of Contents:
The Concept of Alternative Medicine
Defining Alternative Medicine
The History and Evolution
Forms of Alternative Medicine
Herbs and Botanicals
The Power of Herbs
Scientifically-Backed Botanicals
How to Use Herbs Safely
Acupuncture and Acupressure
Understanding Acupuncture
The Science behind Acupressure
Case Studies
Homeopathy
Basics of Homeopathy
Homeopathic Remedies
Criticisms and Controversies
Aromatherapy
Understanding Aromatherapy
Benefits and Uses
Essential Oils Guide
Chiropractic Medicine

An Introduction to Chiropractic Medicine

Pros and Cons

Chiropractic Techniques

Nutrition and Diet Therapy

Nutritional Approach to Health

Diet Therapy Methods

Understanding Food Therapy

Yoga and Meditation

Overview of Yoga

The Science of Meditation

The Mind-Body Connection

Naturopathic Medicine

Principles of Naturopathy

Therapies and Treatments

The Role of a Naturopathic Doctor

Ayurvedic Medicine

Concept of Ayurveda

Ayurvedic Practices

The Three Doshas

Energy Medicine

The Field of Energy Medicine

Techniques and Treatments

Understanding Qi and Meridians

Integrative Medicine

Integrative vs Alternative Medicine

The Scope of Integrative Care

Integrative Medicine Case Studies

Research and Studies on Alternative Medicine
Overview of Studies
Scientifically-Backed Benefits
Current Research in the Field
Risks and Challenges of Alternative Medicine
Understanding the Risks
Ethical Issues
Regulations and Guidelines
The Future of Alternative Medicine
Emerging Trends
Impact on Healthcare System
Personalized Alternative Treatment
Have Questions / Comments?
Get Another Book Free

The Concept of Alternative Medicine

Alternative medicine encompasses a wide range of healing practices that fall outside of conventional, evidence-based medical treatments. These approaches often focus on natural remedies, holistic care, and mind-body connections. Rather than relying solely on pharmaceutical drugs and surgery, alternative medicine tends to prioritize prevention, lifestyle changes, and treatments that aim to restore balance within the body.

One prominent example is acupuncture, an ancient practice rooted in Traditional Chinese Medicine (TCM). It involves inserting thin needles into specific points on the body to stimulate energy flow and encourage the body's natural healing abilities. Research has suggested that acupuncture can help with pain management, stress relief, and even symptoms of anxiety and depression, although its mechanisms are still being studied.

Herbal medicine is another widely practiced form, utilizing plant-based substances to treat a variety of conditions. Many modern pharmaceuticals are derived from plants, so herbal medicine draws on centuries of knowledge about plant compounds. Common herbs like echinacea, ginseng, and peppermint have been used to boost immunity, reduce inflammation, and ease digestive issues. While some herbal remedies have been supported by scientific studies, it is important to consider quality, dosage, and potential side effects, as herbs can interact with other medications.

Homeopathy is based on the principle of "like cures like" and involves using extremely diluted substances to stimulate the body's self-healing abilities. Despite controversy and skepticism in the medical community, some individuals report improvements from homeopathic treatments, particularly for conditions like allergies, colds, and chronic pain.

Chiropractic care focuses on diagnosing and treating mechanical disorders of the musculoskeletal system, particularly the spine. Chiropractors use spinal manipulation to treat a variety of ailments, including back pain, neck pain, and headaches. Research supports its effectiveness for certain conditions, though there is ongoing debate about the extent of its benefits for other health issues.

Massage therapy, which involves manipulating the muscles and soft tissues of the body, is another popular form of alternative treatment. It can relieve muscle tension, improve circulation, and reduce stress. Studies have shown massage therapy to be beneficial for conditions like chronic pain, arthritis, and anxiety.

Mind-body practices, such as yoga and meditation, are also integral parts of alternative medicine. These practices promote mental and emotional well-being by helping individuals achieve greater physical flexibility, reduce stress, and increase mindfulness. Many studies highlight the positive effects of yoga on overall health, including improved cardiovascular function, reduced anxiety, and better posture.

Although alternative medicine is often met with skepticism by mainstream healthcare professionals, it has grown in popularity due to its holistic approach and natural treatment options.

People seek alternative treatments for various reasons, including dissatisfaction with conventional medicine, a desire for fewer side effects, or the appeal of more personalized care. However, it's crucial to approach alternative therapies with discernment and to consult healthcare providers when necessary, as not all alternative treatments are backed by rigorous scientific research. In some cases, unproven methods can cause harm or delay the diagnosis of serious conditions.

Ultimately, the growing interest in alternative medicine reflects a shift toward more patient-centered care, where individuals are looking for treatments that align with their values and beliefs about health. It's essential to remain open to integrating alternative practices alongside conventional treatments when appropriate, ensuring a balanced and informed approach to wellness.

Defining Alternative Medicine

Alternative medicine refers to a broad range of healing practices, treatments, and therapies that fall outside the scope of conventional, evidence-based medical approaches. Often viewed as complementary or an alternative to mainstream healthcare, these practices are grounded in the belief that the body has the inherent ability to heal itself, given the right conditions. Rather than focusing solely on pharmaceutical interventions or surgical procedures, alternative medicine often emphasizes natural remedies, lifestyle changes, and holistic approaches that treat the person as a whole—mind, body, and spirit.

One key aspect of alternative medicine is its emphasis on individualized care. Practitioners often consider a person's lifestyle, emotional well-being, and environmental factors when recommending treatments. This contrasts with traditional medicine, which tends to focus more on treating specific symptoms or diseases. For example, while conventional medicine might treat an illness with prescription drugs, alternative approaches might explore dietary changes, stress management techniques, or herbal supplements as part of a treatment plan.

Common practices within alternative medicine include acupuncture, herbal medicine, homeopathy, and chiropractic care. Acupuncture, a practice rooted in Traditional Chinese

Medicine, involves inserting thin needles into specific points on the body to help balance the flow of energy, or "qi." This technique is often used for pain management and to address conditions like headaches, digestive issues, and stress. Herbal medicine, another widespread alternative therapy, uses plant-based substances to promote healing. Many well-known herbs, such as echinacea and garlic, have been used for centuries for their purported medicinal properties, particularly for boosting the immune system and improving cardiovascular health.

Homeopathy operates on the principle that "like cures like," using highly diluted substances to stimulate the body's healing response. Although its effectiveness remains a subject of debate, homeopathy continues to have a dedicated following, with proponents using it to treat conditions ranging from allergies to anxiety.

Chiropractic care, which focuses on diagnosing and treating musculoskeletal disorders, especially those related to the spine, is another widely practiced form of alternative medicine. Chiropractors use spinal manipulation to address pain and improve mobility. Many people seek chiropractic treatment for back pain, neck pain, and headaches, and some studies suggest that it can be effective for these conditions.

In addition to these physical treatments, alternative medicine also includes mind-body therapies like yoga, meditation, and mindfulness practices. These therapies emphasize the connection between mental and physical health, aiming to reduce stress, improve mental clarity, and enhance overall well-being. For example, yoga combines physical postures, breathing exercises, and meditation to improve flexibility, balance, and relaxation.

While alternative medicine can be appealing to many for its focus on prevention and natural healing, it is important to acknowledge that not all practices are equally supported by scientific research. Some therapies may have limited or inconclusive evidence regarding their effectiveness, and in certain cases, treatments could even be harmful if not properly managed. As a result, those considering alternative therapies should carefully research the methods and consult healthcare professionals to ensure that they are making informed decisions about their health.

Ultimately, alternative medicine offers a diverse and evolving set of practices that cater to individuals seeking different paths to health and wellness. Its holistic focus and integration of natural remedies provide an appealing alternative to conventional medical treatments, but as with all health-related choices, it's crucial to approach these practices thoughtfully and with an open mind.

The History and Evolution

Alternative medicine has roots that stretch back thousands of years, evolving alongside human civilization and often intertwined with cultural beliefs and practices. The early foundations of alternative healing systems were shaped by ancient cultures, each developing their own methods for understanding the human body and treating illness. From the herbal remedies of early societies to the intricate energy systems found in Eastern medicine, alternative practices have been central to health and wellness throughout history.

One of the oldest known forms of alternative medicine is traditional Chinese medicine (TCM), which dates back over 2,000 years. TCM includes practices such as acupuncture, herbal medicine, and dietary therapy, all designed to balance the body's vital energy, or "qi." The principles of TCM suggest that health is achieved when the body's energy flows freely, and disease arises when there is an imbalance or blockage. This holistic approach not only treats physical symptoms but also considers emotional and spiritual well-being.

Similarly, in India, Ayurveda, a system of medicine that originated around 5,000 years ago, emphasizes the balance of the body's three doshas—vata, pitta, and kapha. Ayurveda combines dietary recommendations, herbal treatments, yoga, and meditation to restore harmony within the body and mind. The philosophy behind Ayurveda is that wellness is achieved through a balanced life, and it continues to be practiced widely today, with increasing recognition in the West.

In the West, alternative medicine has also evolved over centuries, drawing influence from the ancient Greek physician Hippocrates, who is often regarded as the "father of medicine." He advocated for the healing power of nature, stressing the importance of diet, exercise, and a balanced lifestyle for maintaining health. However, it wasn't until the rise of the scientific and medical revolutions in Europe, beginning in the 16th century, that Western medicine became more focused on surgery and pharmaceuticals, sidelining many of the traditional healing practices that had been widely used before.

Despite the dominance of conventional medicine in the Western world, alternative practices persisted in various forms. In the 19th century, herbalism and homeopathy gained popularity, with figures like Samuel Hahnemann, the founder of homeopathy, promoting the idea of "like cures like" and the use of highly diluted substances to treat ailments. Homeopathy became a significant alternative treatment, particularly in Europe and North America, despite facing skepticism from the mainstream medical community.

The 20th century saw the rise of chiropractic care and naturopathy. Chiropractic medicine, founded by D.D. Palmer in 1895, emphasized the role of the spine in health and the treatment of musculoskeletal disorders through spinal adjustments. Naturopathy, on the other hand, focused on natural treatments such as nutrition, hydrotherapy, and physical manipulation, promoting the body's ability to heal itself without the use of pharmaceuticals. Both modalities grew in popularity during the early to mid-1900s and continue to be practiced by millions worldwide today.

In more recent decades, the late 20th and early 21st centuries have seen a resurgence in the popularity of alternative medicine, particularly in Western societies. With growing concerns over the side effects and long-term risks of pharmaceutical drugs, many individuals are turning to alternative therapies as a natural, holistic approach to health. Practices such as acupuncture, massage therapy, and yoga have become mainstream, with a greater emphasis on wellness and prevention. This shift can also be attributed to the increasing recognition of the mind-body connection and the desire for treatments that focus not just on alleviating symptoms but on achieving overall balance and well-being.

At the same time, modern scientific advancements have begun to investigate and validate some alternative practices. Acupuncture, for example, has been the subject of numerous studies, and there is mounting evidence supporting its effectiveness in treating pain and certain other conditions. Similarly, the use of herbal medicine is now being studied more rigorously, with many herbs showing promise for a variety of health conditions.

Alternative medicine has evolved significantly over the centuries, and its history reflects the shifting views on health, disease, and the human body. While some practices have faced skepticism and resistance, many have endured and evolved into the widely recognized and practiced therapies we see today. As more people seek alternatives to conventional medical treatments, the future of alternative medicine is likely to continue its growth, integrating ancient wisdom with modern scientific inquiry.

Forms of Alternative Medicine

Alternative medicine encompasses a wide array of practices and therapies that differ from conventional medical treatments. These forms of healing typically focus on natural methods, holistic care, and the body's intrinsic ability to heal itself. Although many alternative therapies are centuries old, they continue to evolve and gain popularity worldwide for their perceived benefits in promoting overall wellness and addressing health conditions without relying heavily on pharmaceuticals or invasive procedures.

Acupuncture, one of the most well-known forms, originated in China over 2,000 years ago and remains a cornerstone of Traditional Chinese Medicine (TCM). It involves inserting thin needles at specific points on the body to stimulate energy flow, or "qi," which is believed to balance the body and promote healing. Modern research has shown that acupuncture can help with pain relief, reduce inflammation, and even alleviate symptoms of stress and anxiety, though its precise mechanisms are still being explored.

Herbal medicine is another significant component of alternative practices. Throughout history, plants have been used for medicinal purposes, and many modern pharmaceuticals are derived from botanical compounds. Herbs like ginseng, echinacea, and peppermint have long been used for their healing properties, targeting everything from immune support to digestive issues. Though herbal medicine has gained widespread use, it is important to approach it with caution, as not all herbal remedies are well-regulated, and some may interact with prescription medications.

Homeopathy, founded by Samuel Hahnemann in the late 18th century, is based on the principle of "like cures like." This practice involves using highly diluted substances that, in larger amounts, would cause symptoms similar to the condition being treated. Despite controversy and skepticism within the medical community, homeopathy continues to be used for a range of ailments, particularly chronic conditions such as allergies, headaches, and digestive disorders. Research into its effectiveness remains mixed, with some studies showing benefits while others question its scientific basis.

Chiropractic care focuses on the musculoskeletal system, particularly the spine, and is often used to treat back pain, neck pain, and headaches. Chiropractors use manual manipulation techniques, most commonly spinal adjustments, to realign the spine and improve the body's function. Research has supported its efficacy in treating certain types of pain, particularly for conditions like lower back pain, though some skeptics argue its effectiveness for more complex health issues.

Naturopathy is a system of medicine that emphasizes natural remedies and the body's ability to heal itself. Naturopaths may recommend a combination of dietary changes, herbal supplements, hydrotherapy, and physical treatments to address a range of health issues. The focus is often on prevention and supporting the body's innate healing processes. Naturopathy has grown in popularity, particularly in North America and Europe, and is commonly used for conditions such as digestive problems, allergies, and chronic fatigue.

Massage therapy is widely used for relaxation and pain relief. This practice involves manipulating the muscles and soft tissues of the body to relieve tension, improve circulation, and reduce stress. It has been shown to be effective in treating conditions like chronic pain, fibromyalgia, and anxiety. Different styles of massage, such as Swedish, deep tissue, and Shiatsu, each offer specific benefits and techniques for promoting healing and relaxation.

Mind-body practices, such as yoga and meditation, have gained immense popularity in recent decades. These therapies focus on the connection between mental and physical health, using practices that promote mindfulness, relaxation, and stress reduction. Yoga, which combines physical postures with breathing exercises and meditation, has been shown to improve flexibility, reduce anxiety, and enhance overall well-being. Meditation, on the other hand, focuses on cultivating mental clarity and emotional balance. Both practices are increasingly integrated into wellness routines as tools for managing stress and improving mental health.

Another growing area within alternative medicine is the use of essential oils in aromatherapy. Essential oils, extracted from plants, are believed to have therapeutic properties when inhaled or applied topically. Lavender, eucalyptus, and peppermint are commonly used to address issues such as stress, insomnia, and respiratory problems. While more research is needed, some studies have shown that aromatherapy can have a positive impact on mood and relaxation.

While alternative medicine is embraced by many for its emphasis on natural treatments and holistic care, it is essential to approach these therapies with care and discernment. Not all alternative practices are backed by extensive scientific research, and some may pose risks if used improperly or in conjunction with conventional treatments. It is always advisable to consult a healthcare provider before pursuing alternative therapies, especially when dealing with serious health conditions.

Herbs and Botanicals

Herbs and botanicals have played a central role in alternative medicine for centuries, with many plants being valued for their healing properties. Across cultures, from ancient civilizations in Egypt, China, and India to modern-day practices, plant-based remedies have been used to treat a variety of conditions, ranging from minor ailments like headaches to more complex chronic diseases. In fact, a significant portion of today's pharmaceutical drugs are derived from plant compounds, underscoring the deep connection between nature and medicine.

One of the most widely used herbs is **Echinacea**, often associated with boosting the immune system. It is commonly used to treat colds and flu, with some studies suggesting that it can reduce the severity and duration of these illnesses. Echinacea is believed to stimulate the body's natural defenses by increasing the production of white blood cells, although more research is needed to fully understand its mechanisms.

Ginseng, another popular herb, is well-known for its ability to enhance energy and combat fatigue. This herb has been used in traditional medicine, particularly in East Asia, for thousands of years. Ginseng is thought to support the body's adaptation to stress and improve mental clarity. It contains active compounds known as ginsenosides, which are believed to have anti-inflammatory and antioxidant effects. However, it is important to note that ginseng can interact with certain medications, so it should be used cautiously under the guidance of a healthcare provider.

Peppermint is another widely used herb, especially for digestive issues. It has been shown to help relieve symptoms of irritable bowel syndrome (IBS), such as bloating and abdominal discomfort. The menthol in peppermint can help relax the muscles of the gastrointestinal tract, promoting smoother digestion. It is also commonly used for headaches and nausea, either through tea or essential oil applications.

Turmeric, renowned for its bright yellow color, has become one of the most popular botanicals in recent years due to its powerful anti-inflammatory properties. The active compound in turmeric, **curcumin**, is thought to inhibit certain enzymes that contribute to inflammation in the body. While turmeric is commonly used in cooking, it is also available in supplement form for those seeking its medicinal benefits, particularly for conditions like arthritis and inflammatory bowel disease.

Lavender, often used for its calming properties, is favored in aromatherapy for promoting relaxation and reducing anxiety. The essential oil of lavender has been shown in studies to decrease symptoms of stress, insomnia, and even mild pain. Lavender's soothing effects extend beyond emotional well-being; it has also been applied topically for skin irritation and minor burns, thanks to its antiseptic qualities.

Chamomile, a gentle herb often consumed as tea, has long been used for its calming effects. Known to promote better sleep and alleviate anxiety, chamomile has also been used for digestive problems like indigestion and bloating. It contains flavonoids that contribute to its anti-inflammatory and sedative effects, making it a popular choice for relaxation and promoting restful sleep.

Garlic, often found in kitchens around the world, is also a powerful medicinal herb. Rich in sulfur compounds, garlic has been used for centuries to combat infections, reduce blood pressure, and support cardiovascular health. Allicin, the compound responsible for garlic's distinctive odor, is believed to contribute to its ability to fight bacteria, lower cholesterol, and improve immune function.

In addition to these well-known herbs, countless other botanicals are valued for their medicinal properties. **Ashwagandha**, a staple of Ayurvedic medicine, is used to reduce stress and improve stamina. **Milk thistle** has been used to support liver function, while **St. John's Wort** is often used as a natural treatment for mild depression. **Ginkgo biloba**, with its potential to improve circulation and cognitive function, is frequently used in cases of memory loss or cognitive decline.

While herbs and botanicals offer promising health benefits, they must be used with caution. Many herbs contain active compounds that can interact with medications, potentially causing side effects or reducing the effectiveness of prescribed treatments. Furthermore, not all herbs are regulated by authorities like the FDA, which can lead to variability in quality and potency across products. As with any form of medicine, it is essential to consult with a healthcare provider before using herbs, especially for individuals with pre-existing health conditions or who are pregnant or breastfeeding.

In conclusion, herbs and botanicals are integral to alternative medicine, offering a wealth of natural remedies for a wide variety of conditions. Their therapeutic properties, ranging from anti-inflammatory effects to immune support, continue to be explored through modern scientific research, further validating their place in holistic health practices. Whether used alone or in combination with other treatments, these plants represent a connection to centuries of natural healing traditions that still resonate today.

The Power of Herbs

Herbs have been revered for their healing properties for thousands of years, playing a significant role in both traditional and alternative medicine. These natural remedies offer a range of therapeutic benefits, from soothing common ailments to supporting complex systems within the body. The power of herbs lies not only in their ability to treat specific conditions but also in their holistic approach, aiming to restore balance and harmony to the body as a whole.

One of the most powerful herbs in alternative medicine is **ginseng**, known for its ability to boost energy levels, reduce fatigue, and enhance overall vitality. Often referred to as an adaptogen, ginseng helps the body adapt to stress by regulating the adrenal glands and supporting immune function. It has been used for centuries in Eastern medicine to improve mental clarity, increase endurance, and support sexual health. While studies have shown promising results for its effectiveness in improving energy levels, it is important to use it with caution, as it can interact with certain medications, particularly those used for blood pressure or diabetes.

Another herb with remarkable healing powers is **turmeric**. The active compound in turmeric, **curcumin**, is celebrated for its potent anti-inflammatory and antioxidant properties. It has been extensively studied for its ability to alleviate pain and reduce inflammation, making it particularly useful for conditions like arthritis, joint pain, and inflammatory bowel disease. Turmeric also plays a role in supporting liver function and protecting against oxidative stress, helping to prevent cellular damage caused by free radicals. Many people add turmeric to their diet through cooking, but supplements and teas are also commonly used to harness its medicinal benefits.

Peppermint is another herb known for its therapeutic qualities, particularly in promoting digestive health. The menthol in peppermint has a calming effect on the muscles of the gastrointestinal tract, helping to relieve symptoms of bloating, gas, and indigestion. It is also effective in treating irritable bowel syndrome (IBS), with studies suggesting that peppermint oil can reduce abdominal pain and discomfort. In addition to its digestive benefits, peppermint has antimicrobial properties that can help soothe sore throats and alleviate headaches.

For stress relief and mental well-being, **lavender** has long been used in aromatherapy. Lavender essential oil is often diffused to calm the nervous system, reduce anxiety, and improve sleep quality. Research has shown that lavender has a direct effect on the brain's neurotransmitters, helping to lower cortisol levels and promote relaxation. It is also used topically to treat minor burns, cuts, and skin irritations due to its antiseptic properties. Whether used as an oil, tea, or in its dried form, lavender remains one of the most popular herbs for promoting emotional balance and relaxation.

Echinacea is a well-known herb for supporting the immune system, particularly in the treatment and prevention of colds and flu. Echinacea contains compounds that stimulate the production of white blood cells, which are essential for fighting off infections. Many people use it at the onset of a cold to reduce symptoms and shorten the duration of the illness. Although research on echinacea's effectiveness is still ongoing, many studies support its ability to strengthen immune function and provide relief from common respiratory infections.

Garlic is another herb with a broad range of health benefits, particularly for cardiovascular health. The sulfur compounds found in garlic, particularly **allicin**, are known to lower cholesterol levels, reduce blood pressure, and improve circulation. Garlic also has antimicrobial properties, making it effective in fighting off infections and supporting overall immune health. Regular consumption of garlic has been linked to a reduced risk of heart disease, and its potential to protect against certain types of cancer is also being actively researched.

Chamomile, widely consumed as a calming tea, is another herb with powerful effects on the body and mind. Known for its soothing properties, chamomile is often used to alleviate insomnia, reduce anxiety, and promote relaxation. The flavonoids in chamomile have anti-inflammatory and antioxidant effects, making it beneficial for conditions like digestive discomfort and skin irritations. Chamomile's gentle nature makes it a popular herb for both children and adults seeking natural remedies for stress or sleep-related issues.

The healing power of herbs is not just in their active compounds, but in their ability to work synergistically with the body's natural processes. When used appropriately, herbs can support the body's immune system, reduce inflammation, improve circulation, and enhance mental clarity. Many herbs also provide nutritional benefits, offering vitamins, minerals, and antioxidants that contribute to overall health.

However, it is important to approach herbal remedies with care. While herbs are natural, they can still cause side effects or interact with medications, especially if used incorrectly or in excessive amounts. For instance, **St. John's Wort**, commonly used to treat mild depression, can interfere with the effectiveness of various prescription medications, including birth control and blood thinners. As with any form of medicine, it is essential to consult with a healthcare provider before starting herbal treatments, particularly if you have existing health conditions or are on medication.

In conclusion, herbs offer a powerful, natural way to support health and well-being. From enhancing digestion to promoting relaxation, the wide variety of healing plants available today continues to be an essential component of alternative medicine. Whether used in teas, supplements, or as essential oils, these botanical remedies have stood the test of time for their therapeutic benefits and continue to provide holistic care for people seeking to improve their health naturally.

Scientifically-Backed Botanicals

In recent years, scientific research has increasingly supported the use of certain botanicals in alternative medicine, validating traditional healing practices with evidence-based findings. Many herbs and plant-based compounds, once used primarily in folk medicine, are now being recognized for their therapeutic properties. These botanicals, backed by modern science, are showing promise for treating a wide range of health conditions, from inflammation to anxiety, and even chronic diseases like diabetes and cardiovascular disorders.

One of the most studied botanicals is **turmeric**, particularly its active compound **curcumin**. Known for its potent anti-inflammatory and antioxidant properties, curcumin has been shown in numerous studies to help reduce symptoms of conditions like arthritis, inflammatory bowel disease, and even heart disease. Research has also explored its role in cancer prevention, with some studies suggesting that curcumin may inhibit the growth of cancer cells and enhance the effectiveness of certain chemotherapy treatments. Despite the promising research, curcumin's bioavailability—how well the body absorbs it—remains a topic of discussion, with studies exploring ways to enhance its absorption for better effectiveness.

Echinacea, often used to combat colds and flu, has also gained attention from the scientific community. Various studies have shown that echinacea can stimulate the immune system, enhancing the body's ability to fight off infections. While some studies report mixed results regarding its effectiveness in preventing or reducing the duration of colds, many experts agree that it may help with the severity and duration of symptoms when taken at the onset of illness. The active compounds in echinacea, such as alkamides and polysaccharides, are believed to play a crucial role in its immune-boosting effects, although more research is needed to fully understand its mechanisms.

Ginseng, another widely studied herb, has been shown to improve energy, mental clarity, and immune function. Research supports its use as an adaptogen, meaning it helps the body adapt to stress and restore balance. Ginseng has been shown to have positive effects on physical performance and endurance, and there is growing evidence of its ability to improve cognitive function, particularly in aging individuals. The active compounds in ginseng, called ginsenosides, have been shown to have anti-inflammatory, antioxidant, and neuroprotective effects, making it a promising option for those seeking natural ways to combat fatigue, improve concentration, and boost overall vitality.

Peppermint is another herb with significant scientific backing, particularly for its ability to improve digestive health. Studies have shown that peppermint oil can relieve symptoms of irritable bowel syndrome (IBS), such as bloating, cramping, and diarrhea. The menthol in peppermint has been shown to relax the muscles of the gastrointestinal tract, easing discomfort and promoting smoother digestion. Additionally, peppermint's antimicrobial properties make it effective in treating issues like sore throats and respiratory congestion.

Garlic, widely known for its cardiovascular benefits, is also supported by scientific research. Allicin, the active compound in garlic, has been shown to reduce blood pressure, lower cholesterol levels, and improve circulation. Studies suggest that regular garlic consumption may reduce the risk of heart disease and stroke by improving lipid profiles and preventing the formation of arterial plaque. Garlic's antibacterial and antifungal properties also contribute to its role in supporting the immune system and preventing infections.

Lavender, with its calming effects, has been extensively studied for its role in reducing anxiety, improving sleep quality, and promoting relaxation. Clinical studies have shown that lavender essential oil can have a significant impact on stress levels, with aromatherapy sessions leading to reduced anxiety and improved mood. In fact, a study published in the *Journal of Clinical Psychiatry* found that lavender oil capsules were as effective as lorazepam, a prescription medication, in treating generalized anxiety disorder. Additionally, lavender's ability to promote better sleep has been confirmed in various studies, making it a popular choice for individuals struggling with insomnia or disrupted sleep cycles.

St. John's Wort, long used for its antidepressant effects, has also been the subject of scientific scrutiny. Several clinical trials have shown that St. John's Wort can be effective in treating mild to moderate depression. The active compounds in St. John's Wort, particularly hypericin and hyperforin, are believed to affect the brain's serotonin levels, similar to the way pharmaceutical antidepressants work. However, St. John's Wort is known to interact with a number of medications, including birth control and blood thinners, so it should be used cautiously and under the supervision of a healthcare provider.

Ashwagandha, an adaptogenic herb used in Ayurvedic medicine, has garnered scientific interest for its ability to reduce stress and improve mental health. Studies have shown that ashwagandha can lower cortisol levels, the hormone responsible for stress, and improve the body's ability to cope with stress. In addition to its stress-reducing properties, ashwagandha has been shown to improve cognitive function, support immune health, and even enhance physical performance. The herb's wide range of benefits makes it a popular choice for individuals seeking natural ways to improve their overall well-being.

Milk thistle, commonly used to support liver health, contains a compound called **silymarin**, which has been shown to protect liver cells from damage and promote liver regeneration. Research has confirmed that silymarin can be beneficial in treating liver conditions such as fatty liver disease, hepatitis, and cirrhosis. Studies suggest that milk thistle's antioxidant properties help reduce inflammation in the liver, supporting overall liver function and detoxification.

These scientifically backed botanicals illustrate the growing body of evidence supporting the therapeutic potential of plants in alternative medicine. While further research is needed to fully understand the mechanisms behind many of these herbs, the existing studies highlight their effectiveness in supporting health and treating various conditions. When used properly, under the guidance of a healthcare provider, these botanicals offer a natural, scientifically supported approach to health and wellness.

How to Use Herbs Safely

Herbs have been used for centuries as natural remedies, offering a wide range of benefits for physical and mental well-being. However, like any form of treatment, it is important to use herbs safely to maximize their effectiveness and minimize potential risks. Proper knowledge of dosages, potential interactions, and proper preparation methods can ensure that herbal remedies provide their intended benefits without causing harm.

One of the first steps in using herbs safely is to understand their appropriate dosage. Herbs are potent, and the correct dosage can vary based on the specific herb, the method of administration, and the individual's age, health condition, and other factors. For instance, while an herbal tea made from chamomile flowers may require only a few grams of dried flowers per cup, concentrated extracts or supplements may require much smaller doses. Overuse of certain herbs, such as **ginseng** or **turmeric**, can lead to adverse effects like digestive upset or increased risk of bleeding. It's essential to follow the dosage recommendations provided by reputable sources or consult a healthcare provider for guidance.

Another critical aspect of using herbs safely is understanding potential interactions with prescription medications or other treatments. Some herbs can interfere with the action of prescription drugs, either diminishing their effectiveness or causing harmful side effects. For example, **St. John's Wort**, often used for mild depression, can reduce the effectiveness of birth control pills, anticoagulants, and certain antidepressants. Similarly, **garlic** in high amounts can increase the risk of bleeding when combined with blood thinners like warfarin. Always inform your healthcare provider about any herbs or supplements you are taking to ensure there are no harmful interactions with other medications.

When using herbs for medicinal purposes, it is essential to choose high-quality products. Many herbs are available in various forms, including dried leaves, teas, tinctures, extracts, and capsules. However, not all products are created equal. Herbal supplements are not strictly regulated in some countries, and the potency or purity of the product may vary. To reduce the risk of contamination or mislabeling, choose products from reputable manufacturers that have undergone independent testing for quality, potency, and purity. Look for certifications such as organic or third-party testing to ensure the product's authenticity.

One of the safest ways to incorporate herbs into your routine is by using them in a mild, non-invasive form like herbal teas. Teas are easy to prepare and generally considered safe when consumed in moderation. For example, **peppermint** tea can be soothing for digestive issues, while **chamomile** tea is often used to promote relaxation and aid sleep. Drinking herbal teas also provides an opportunity to monitor how your body responds to a particular herb and adjust the amount consumed based on your individual needs.

For more concentrated forms, like herbal extracts or essential oils, it is essential to follow usage guidelines carefully. Essential oils, for example, should never be ingested without professional supervision, as they are highly concentrated and can cause harm if used improperly. If using essential oils for aromatherapy or topical application, always dilute the oil with a carrier oil, like coconut or jojoba oil, to prevent skin irritation or allergic reactions. Perform a patch test on a small area of skin to check for sensitivity before applying the oil to larger areas.

Pregnant or breastfeeding women, as well as individuals with certain health conditions, should exercise extra caution when using herbs. Some herbs can affect hormone levels, cause uterine contractions, or interfere with the development of a fetus. For example, **aloe vera** and **licorice root** should be avoided during pregnancy due to potential risks. Likewise, herbs like **ginger** can be beneficial for nausea but should be used in moderation to avoid potential risks in high doses during pregnancy. Always consult a healthcare provider before using any herb if you are pregnant, breastfeeding, or have a chronic health condition.

Starting with small doses and gradually increasing them is a good practice, particularly if you are new to using herbal remedies. This allows your body to adjust and helps identify any adverse reactions early on. Monitoring how you feel after using a particular herb is essential—if you experience any unusual symptoms like dizziness, headaches, nausea, or allergic reactions, it's important to discontinue use and consult a healthcare provider immediately.

Lastly, sourcing herbs from reliable and ethical suppliers is vital to ensuring their safety. Some herbs are subject to contamination by heavy metals, pesticides, or other harmful substances, so it is essential to purchase from trusted sources that adhere to safety and environmental standards. Wildcrafted herbs, which are harvested from their natural environment, should be collected in areas free of pollutants and pesticides.

In conclusion, herbs can be a safe and effective form of alternative medicine when used properly. By understanding appropriate dosages, recognizing potential interactions, choosing high-quality products, and practicing moderation, you can maximize the benefits of herbal remedies while minimizing risks. Always remember to consult with a healthcare provider, particularly if you are pregnant, breastfeeding, or taking prescription medications, to ensure safe and effective use of herbs in your wellness routine.

Acupuncture and Acupressure

Acupuncture and acupressure are two closely related therapeutic practices that have been integral to traditional Chinese medicine (TCM) for thousands of years. Both techniques are based on the principle that the body's energy, or **qi** (pronounced "chee"), flows through specific pathways, or meridians. When this energy is blocked or unbalanced, it can lead to illness or discomfort. Both acupuncture and acupressure aim to restore the flow of qi, promoting healing and overall well-being by stimulating specific points on the body.

Acupuncture involves the insertion of very fine needles into predetermined points on the body. These needles are strategically placed along the body's meridians, which correspond to different organ systems and physical functions. Acupuncture practitioners believe that by stimulating these points, they can unblock or rebalance the flow of qi, thus alleviating pain and addressing various health conditions. Acupuncture is widely used to treat conditions such as chronic pain (back pain, osteoarthritis, and migraines), stress, digestive issues, and even anxiety and depression.

Research into acupuncture has gained significant traction in recent decades, and there is mounting evidence supporting its effectiveness for a variety of conditions. Multiple studies have shown that acupuncture can significantly reduce pain and improve mobility, particularly in cases of musculoskeletal pain, such as chronic back pain or knee osteoarthritis. Acupuncture has also been linked to improvements in mental health, with studies suggesting that it can reduce anxiety, alleviate symptoms of depression, and even help with insomnia. The exact mechanisms behind acupuncture are still not fully understood, but some theories suggest that the needles stimulate the body's nervous system, triggering the release of endorphins (natural painkillers) and influencing the body's natural healing processes.

Acupressure, on the other hand, is a similar practice, but instead of needles, it involves applying pressure to specific points on the body using the fingers, thumbs, or palms. Acupressure is often considered a more accessible form of acupuncture, as it does not require specialized training or equipment. The same points that are targeted in acupuncture are used in acupressure, and the goal is to release tension, alleviate pain, and promote healing by applying varying degrees of pressure to these points. Acupressure is commonly used for self-care, as individuals can apply it to themselves or with the help of a partner to relieve tension and stress.

One of the most well-known uses of acupressure is for the relief of nausea, particularly in cases of motion sickness or morning sickness during pregnancy. The **P6 point**, located on the inner forearm near the wrist, is a popular acupressure point used to alleviate nausea. Studies have shown that applying gentle pressure to this point can effectively reduce nausea and vomiting, making acupressure a widely used complementary therapy for pregnant women or those undergoing chemotherapy.

Both acupuncture and acupressure are often employed for their ability to reduce stress and promote relaxation. Acupressure can be used to relieve tension headaches, shoulder pain, and muscle stiffness, while acupuncture is often used to treat a broader range of conditions, from chronic pain to stress-related disorders. Many patients who use acupuncture report a sense of calm and deep relaxation during and after treatment, likely due to the stimulation of the body's parasympathetic nervous system, which is responsible for rest and digestion.

The effectiveness of both acupuncture and acupressure is supported by a growing body of scientific research, although there is still some debate in the medical community about their mechanisms. Some researchers suggest that acupuncture may stimulate the release of neurotransmitters like endorphins, which help reduce pain and promote a sense of well-being. Others propose that acupuncture may have a direct effect on the nervous system, improving blood flow and promoting tissue healing. Similarly, acupressure may work by activating the body's pressure receptors, which can trigger the release of pain-relieving chemicals and reduce muscle tension.

Despite their benefits, both acupuncture and acupressure are not suitable for everyone, and certain precautions should be taken. Acupuncture should only be performed by a licensed and trained practitioner to ensure that the needles are inserted safely and correctly. Infections or injury can occur if acupuncture is performed improperly, so it is important to choose a qualified practitioner. Acupressure, while generally safe for most people, should be avoided if there are open wounds, inflammation, or infection in the targeted areas. As with any form of alternative medicine, it is essential to consult with a healthcare provider before starting acupuncture or acupressure, particularly if you are pregnant, have a chronic health condition, or are on medication.

Both acupuncture and acupressure provide valuable alternative therapies that can complement conventional medical treatments, offering relief from a variety of conditions. Whether used to address physical discomfort, mental health concerns, or promote relaxation, these ancient practices continue to be a popular choice for those seeking a natural, holistic approach to health and well-being.

Understanding Acupuncture

Acupuncture is a therapeutic practice rooted in traditional Chinese medicine (TCM) that has gained widespread acceptance worldwide. It involves inserting thin, sterile needles into specific points on the body to stimulate the flow of **qi** (pronounced "chee"), the body's vital energy. The goal of acupuncture is to balance the flow of energy, restore health, and promote healing. While it has been practiced for thousands of years, modern research has provided increasing evidence of its effectiveness in treating a wide range of physical and emotional health conditions.

At the core of acupuncture is the belief that energy flows through the body along pathways known as **meridians**. These meridians are like invisible channels that carry qi to various organs and tissues. When the flow of qi is blocked or imbalanced, it is thought to lead to illness, pain, or other health problems. By inserting needles at specific points along these meridians, acupuncture practitioners aim to restore harmony and improve the body's natural ability to heal.

Acupuncture is used to treat a variety of conditions, ranging from chronic pain to digestive issues, respiratory disorders, and even mental health problems like anxiety and depression. One of the most common uses of acupuncture is for pain management. Conditions such as **back pain, arthritis, migraines**, and **neck pain** can be alleviated through acupuncture treatments. Research has shown that acupuncture can stimulate the body's production of endorphins, which are natural painkillers, as well as other neurotransmitters that help reduce inflammation and promote healing.

In addition to its role in pain relief, acupuncture has been studied for its effectiveness in treating other conditions, such as **insomnia**, **digestive disorders**, and **stress-related ailments**. Acupuncture may promote relaxation and improve sleep by stimulating the release of chemicals that regulate mood and anxiety. Studies have also indicated that acupuncture can help alleviate symptoms of **irritable bowel syndrome (IBS)**, such as bloating, abdominal pain, and irregular bowel movements, by improving digestion and reducing inflammation.

Acupuncture's ability to support mental health has also gained attention in recent years. Many individuals seek acupuncture to help manage **stress, anxiety**, and **depression**. By stimulating certain acupuncture points, the treatment may balance the body's stress response and improve overall emotional well-being. Some studies have suggested that acupuncture may increase the production of **serotonin** and **dopamine**, neurotransmitters that play a key role in mood regulation.

The practice of acupuncture is tailored to the individual. A trained practitioner will first perform an assessment to understand the patient's condition, including lifestyle, diet, emotional health, and physical symptoms. Based on this assessment, the practitioner will select specific acupuncture points to target in the treatment. The needles used are extremely fine and are typically inserted only a few millimeters into the skin. Many people experience little to no pain during the process, and some even report a feeling of deep relaxation during treatment.

Acupuncture is generally considered safe when performed by a licensed and trained practitioner. It is important to ensure that the practitioner follows proper hygiene practices, using sterilized needles to prevent infection. Although acupuncture is non-invasive, it can still have side effects, such as mild bruising, soreness, or lightheadedness, particularly after the first treatment. These effects are usually temporary and subside quickly.

One of the advantages of acupuncture is that it can complement other forms of treatment. It is commonly used alongside conventional medicine for chronic pain, rehabilitation, and stress management, providing a holistic approach to healthcare. In fact, acupuncture has been integrated into some mainstream healthcare settings, such as pain management clinics and rehabilitation centers, for its ability to support recovery and enhance well-being.

Despite its long history, acupuncture's mechanisms of action are still being explored. While there is growing evidence supporting its effectiveness, the scientific community continues to study how acupuncture works at a physiological level. Some theories suggest that acupuncture stimulates the nervous system, triggering the release of chemicals that regulate pain and inflammation. Others propose that acupuncture helps to improve blood circulation and activate the body's healing processes by promoting the flow of energy through the meridians.

Although acupuncture has shown positive results for many individuals, it may not be suitable for everyone. People with certain conditions, such as blood clotting disorders or those who are pregnant, should consult a healthcare provider before starting acupuncture. Additionally, acupuncture should never be used as a substitute for emergency medical care, especially for serious health conditions like heart attacks or strokes.

In conclusion, acupuncture offers a natural and holistic approach to health that can effectively address a variety of physical and emotional conditions. By restoring balance to the body's energy flow, acupuncture helps to promote healing and enhance well-being. As research continues to validate its benefits, acupuncture remains an increasingly popular choice for those seeking alternative treatments to complement conventional medicine.

The Science behind Acupressure

Acupressure is an alternative therapy rooted in traditional Chinese medicine that involves applying manual pressure to specific points on the body, known as acupoints. These acupoints correspond to pathways, or meridians, that are believed to carry vital energy, or **qi**, throughout the body. By stimulating these points, acupressure aims to restore the balance of energy, improve circulation, relieve pain, and promote overall well-being. While acupressure shares similarities with acupuncture, which uses needles, it relies solely on physical pressure, making it an accessible and non-invasive therapy.

The science behind acupressure is still being explored, but several mechanisms have been proposed to explain how it works. One widely accepted theory is that applying pressure to specific points on the body activates the **nervous system**, triggering the release of neurotransmitters like **endorphins** and **serotonin**. Endorphins, known as the body's natural painkillers, are believed to help alleviate pain and promote feelings of relaxation and well-being. Serotonin plays a role in regulating mood, which is why acupressure is often used to help with stress, anxiety, and depression.

Acupressure is thought to influence both the **sympathetic** and **parasympathetic** branches of the autonomic nervous system. The sympathetic nervous system is responsible for the body's "fight-or-flight" response, while the parasympathetic system is linked to the "rest-and-digest" functions. By stimulating certain acupoints, acupressure helps activate the parasympathetic system, promoting relaxation and reducing the effects of stress. This balance is key to improving overall health, as chronic stress can lead to a variety of health problems, including digestive issues, high blood pressure, and weakened immune function.

In addition to stimulating the nervous system, acupressure may also enhance **circulation** by improving blood flow to the targeted areas of the body. This increased circulation can help deliver oxygen and nutrients to tissues, promote healing, and remove metabolic waste products. For example, applying pressure to the **LI4 point** (located between the thumb and index finger) is believed to promote circulation, relieve headaches, and alleviate tension.

The concept of acupressure also involves **reflexology**, which suggests that certain points on the body correspond to organs or systems in the body. For instance, acupressure on the feet or hands is often used to treat symptoms in other parts of the body, such as headaches, digestive problems, or muscle tension. By stimulating these points, acupressure is thought to balance the energy in those specific organs, supporting their function and promoting overall health.

Research into the scientific efficacy of acupressure has shown promising results, particularly for pain management, stress reduction, and nausea relief. Studies have demonstrated that acupressure can significantly reduce pain associated with conditions like **osteoarthritis**, **muscle pain**, and **headaches**. It has also been shown to reduce the severity of **nausea**, especially in cases of motion sickness, chemotherapy, and morning sickness during pregnancy. One of the most widely studied acupressure points is **P6**, located on the inner forearm, which is frequently used to alleviate nausea and vomiting.

In addition to its effectiveness for pain and nausea, acupressure has also been shown to reduce **muscle tension** and improve **sleep quality**. Applying pressure to certain acupoints, such as those on the neck or shoulders, can help relieve muscle tightness and improve flexibility. For individuals struggling with insomnia, acupressure can stimulate relaxation responses, making it easier to fall asleep and stay asleep.

While acupressure is generally considered safe, it is important to note that it may not be suitable for everyone. People with certain medical conditions, such as **blood clotting disorders** or **skin conditions**, should consult with a healthcare provider before using acupressure. Pregnant women, in particular, should avoid certain acupoints that are believed to induce labor or affect pregnancy. As with any form of alternative therapy, it is crucial to seek professional guidance to ensure that acupressure is appropriate for your specific needs and conditions.

In conclusion, the science behind acupressure suggests that this ancient practice can have a significant impact on health by stimulating the nervous system, improving circulation, and balancing energy within the body. By harnessing the body's natural ability to heal, acupressure offers a non-invasive and accessible treatment for a variety of physical and emotional conditions. Although more research is needed to fully understand the mechanisms behind acupressure, the growing body of evidence supporting its effectiveness makes it a promising tool in the realm of alternative medicine.

Case Studies

Case studies in alternative medicine provide valuable insights into the effectiveness of various treatments in real-world settings. These case studies often highlight how individuals have benefited from therapies that fall outside the realm of conventional medicine, offering a deeper understanding of how alternative approaches can complement traditional treatments. While these case studies are not meant to replace rigorous clinical trials, they provide compelling anecdotal evidence and may serve as a starting point for further research into the potential benefits of alternative therapies.

One example of a successful case study involves the use of **acupuncture** for pain management. A 55-year-old woman suffering from chronic back pain, which had been unresponsive to medications and physical therapy, sought acupuncture treatment. After a series of sessions, she reported significant reductions in pain and increased mobility. In this case, acupuncture helped alleviate pain by stimulating the body's natural healing mechanisms, leading to improved circulation and the release of endorphins. This case suggests that acupuncture can be an effective option for individuals with chronic pain who have not found relief through conventional treatments.

Another notable case study comes from the use of **herbal medicine** for managing symptoms of **irritable bowel syndrome (IBS)**. A 40-year-old man with a long history of IBS symptoms, including bloating, abdominal pain, and irregular bowel movements, turned to herbal remedies after conventional medications failed to provide lasting relief. He began using a combination of **peppermint oil** and **ginger supplements**, both of which are known for their digestive benefits. Within weeks, the patient experienced a noticeable reduction in symptoms, including fewer flare-ups and improved digestion. This case highlights the potential of herbal medicine to provide relief for digestive disorders, particularly when traditional treatments are ineffective.

In the realm of **chiropractic care**, a case study of a 30-year-old woman with recurring **migraine headaches** demonstrates how spinal adjustments can help alleviate chronic pain. The patient had been suffering from migraines for years, often leading to days of missed work and decreased quality of life. After several chiropractic treatments, which focused on aligning the cervical spine, the frequency and intensity of her migraines decreased significantly. She reported fewer episodes of migraine pain, and her overall well-being improved. This case supports the theory that chiropractic care may play a role in managing certain types of headaches, particularly those related to spinal misalignments.

Yoga therapy has also been explored through case studies, especially in managing **mental health** conditions like anxiety and depression. A 45-year-old man dealing with high levels of anxiety and stress, compounded by work-related pressure, turned to yoga as a means of managing his mental health. After practicing yoga regularly for several months, he reported feeling less anxious, more centered, and better able to cope with daily stresses. His physical health also improved, with greater flexibility and reduced muscle tension. This case study demonstrates how yoga can benefit not only physical health but also mental well-being, offering a holistic approach to managing stress and anxiety.

A compelling case study of **aromatherapy** involved a 60-year-old woman with **chronic insomnia**. After trying various conventional sleep aids with limited success, she sought alternative methods and turned to aromatherapy using **lavender essential oil**. She began using a diffuser with lavender oil in her bedroom before bedtime. Over the course of several weeks, she experienced improvements in sleep quality and found it easier to fall asleep and stay asleep throughout the night. This case suggests that aromatherapy, specifically the use of lavender, can help individuals struggling with sleep disturbances by promoting relaxation and reducing anxiety.

Homeopathy has also been the subject of several case studies, although its efficacy remains a topic of debate. One case involved a 35-year-old woman who had been struggling with **allergic rhinitis** for years. Despite trying antihistamines and other conventional treatments, her symptoms, including sneezing and nasal congestion, persisted. After receiving a homeopathic remedy tailored to her specific symptoms, she reported a significant improvement, with fewer episodes of sneezing and a reduction in nasal congestion. While more rigorous research is needed to support homeopathy's effectiveness, this case highlights its potential as an alternative treatment for allergies.

Massage therapy is another area where case studies have shown positive results. A case study involving a 50-year-old woman with **fibromyalgia** demonstrated how regular massage therapy could provide relief from chronic pain. The patient had been experiencing widespread muscle pain, fatigue, and sleep disturbances. After receiving consistent deep tissue massages, she reported a significant reduction in pain and muscle stiffness, as well as improved sleep quality. This case provides evidence that massage therapy may be beneficial for individuals suffering from fibromyalgia and other chronic pain conditions.

While these case studies illustrate the potential benefits of various alternative therapies, it is important to remember that individual responses to treatment can vary. Alternative therapies, while promising, are not a one-size-fits-all solution and should be considered as part of an overall wellness plan. In many cases, these treatments work best in conjunction with conventional medical care. It is always advisable to consult a healthcare provider before beginning any alternative treatment, particularly if there are underlying health conditions or ongoing medical treatments.

In conclusion, case studies in alternative medicine offer valuable insights into the real-world effectiveness of treatments like acupuncture, herbal remedies, chiropractic care, yoga, and more. These individual success stories not only highlight the potential benefits of alternative therapies but also encourage further exploration and research into their applications for a variety of health conditions. While not a substitute for scientific clinical trials, these case studies can inspire individuals to consider alternative medicine as part of a holistic approach to health.

Homeopathy

Homeopathy is an alternative medicine system that has sparked both interest and controversy since its creation in the late 18th century by Samuel Hahnemann, a German physician. Based on the principle of "like cures like," homeopathy involves using highly diluted substances to treat symptoms. The central tenet of homeopathy is that a substance that causes symptoms in a healthy person can, in a diluted form, treat similar symptoms in someone who is ill. This theory is grounded in the idea that the body has an inherent ability to heal itself when properly stimulated.

The process of creating homeopathic remedies is unique and involves a method of **potentization**, where substances are diluted and then vigorously shaken, often hundreds of times. This process is believed to enhance the healing properties of the remedy while minimizing the toxic effects of the substance. The final product typically contains no molecules of the original substance, leading some critics to argue that homeopathic remedies may be no more effective than placebos. Despite this, millions of people worldwide continue to use homeopathy as a treatment for a range of ailments, from minor conditions like colds to chronic illnesses.

Homeopathy is based on two main principles: **similars** (the idea that a substance that causes symptoms in a healthy person can cure those same symptoms in a sick person) and **minimal dose** (the idea that the lower the dose, the greater the effect). Proponents of homeopathy believe that remedies work by stimulating the body's vital force, a life energy that regulates health. According to this belief, illness occurs when the vital force is out of balance, and homeopathic treatments help restore that balance, allowing the body to heal itself.

A key concept in homeopathy is the use of **individualized treatment**. Homeopaths take a detailed history of a patient's physical, emotional, and psychological state, seeking patterns that reveal the underlying cause of illness. This approach differs from conventional medicine, which often focuses on specific diseases or symptoms. Homeopathic practitioners believe that by addressing the whole person—rather than just targeting a disease or condition—they can bring about a more lasting and effective cure.

Homeopathic remedies are made from a wide variety of substances, including plant extracts, minerals, and animal products. For example, **Arnica montana**, a common homeopathic remedy, is made from the mountain daisy and is often used to treat bruising, muscle soreness, and trauma. Another popular remedy, **Oscillococcinum**, is made from duck liver and heart and is often used to treat flu-like symptoms. While these substances are highly diluted, the belief in homeopathy is that their energetic imprint remains, providing therapeutic benefits despite the absence of the original material.

While homeopathy is widely used by millions of people, particularly for conditions like colds, allergies, and insomnia, it remains a topic of debate. Scientific research on homeopathy has yielded mixed results. Some studies suggest that homeopathy may offer benefits for specific conditions, while others have found no greater effect than a placebo. This has led to heated discussions within the medical community about whether homeopathic treatments are truly effective or if the benefits seen by patients are due to the placebo effect or natural recovery.

Despite the controversy, many people report positive outcomes from homeopathic treatments, particularly in cases where conventional medicine has proven ineffective or where patients seek a more holistic approach. For example, homeopathy has been used as a complementary treatment for chronic conditions such as asthma, eczema, and rheumatoid arthritis. Supporters of homeopathy argue that it is a safe, non-invasive option for those looking for an alternative to pharmaceutical drugs, especially since homeopathic remedies are generally considered to have few side effects when taken as directed.

One of the major criticisms of homeopathy is that it lacks a scientific explanation for how extremely diluted remedies can have an effect. The molecular dilution often goes beyond the point where any molecules of the original substance remain, raising questions about how such remedies could work. Despite this, homeopathy has a long-standing history, and its use continues to be widespread. Many homeopaths and patients believe that it offers a valuable approach to health care, particularly for those seeking natural or individualized treatments.

In conclusion, homeopathy is a form of alternative medicine that focuses on treating individuals rather than diseases, using highly diluted substances to stimulate the body's healing processes. While it has been subject to scientific scrutiny and remains controversial in the medical community, many individuals turn to homeopathy for its individualized approach and its use in treating a variety of health concerns. Whether or not it is scientifically proven, homeopathy continues to be a widely practiced and cherished treatment for many people around the world.

Basics of Homeopathy

Homeopathy is an alternative healing system that operates on the principle of **"like cures like,"** which means that a substance capable of causing symptoms in a healthy person can, in a highly diluted form, treat similar symptoms in a sick person. This foundational concept was developed by Samuel Hahnemann, a German physician, in the late 18th century. The idea is based on the belief that the body has an inherent ability to heal itself when stimulated appropriately, and that this healing can be guided by using remedies made from natural substances that match the patient's symptoms.

The process of creating homeopathic remedies involves **potentization**, where the original substance (whether plant, mineral, or animal-based) is diluted in a series of steps and then vigorously shaken or "succussed." This procedure is said to enhance the healing properties of the remedy while reducing any harmful effects. The final solution is typically so diluted that it often contains no molecules of the original substance, which has led to debate over whether homeopathic remedies have any pharmacological activity or if they work purely through the placebo effect.

One of the key principles of homeopathy is **individualization**. Rather than simply diagnosing a disease and matching it with a one-size-fits-all remedy, homeopathy takes into account the entire person. This includes not only the physical symptoms but also emotional, mental, and lifestyle factors. Homeopaths believe that treating the whole person—not just the illness—

restores balance and allows the body to heal naturally. A remedy is selected based on the patient's unique symptoms, personality traits, and even life experiences.

Homeopathic remedies are used for a wide range of conditions, from minor ailments like **headaches**, **insomnia**, and **common colds**, to more chronic conditions such as **eczema**, **asthma**, and **rheumatoid arthritis**. Some of the most well-known remedies include **Arnica montana**, often used to treat bruising and muscle soreness, and **Apis mellifica**, made from the venom of honeybees and commonly used for swelling and allergic reactions.

The effectiveness of homeopathy remains controversial in the scientific community. Critics argue that because homeopathic remedies are so diluted, they likely do not contain any measurable active ingredients, and thus cannot produce the claimed therapeutic effects. However, proponents of homeopathy argue that the remedies work by influencing the body's vital energy, or **life force**, in a way that conventional medicine does not. Some studies have shown positive effects, especially in the treatment of pain, anxiety, and various chronic conditions, but the overall body of research remains inconclusive.

Despite skepticism from many in the medical field, homeopathy continues to be popular worldwide. Many people turn to it as a natural and gentle alternative to conventional medicine, particularly when looking for solutions for chronic conditions or when seeking to avoid the side effects of pharmaceutical drugs. Since homeopathic remedies are made from natural substances and highly diluted, they are generally considered safe when used appropriately, with few side effects or risks when administered under the guidance of a trained homeopath.

One of the most attractive aspects of homeopathy is its holistic approach. It does not treat diseases in isolation but rather considers the interplay of the physical, emotional, and mental aspects of health. In this way, homeopathy emphasizes preventive care and wellness, encouraging individuals to maintain balance in all areas of their lives.

For those interested in homeopathy, it is important to work with a trained and experienced practitioner who can tailor treatments to the individual. While homeopathy is widely used as a complementary therapy alongside conventional treatments, it is important to discuss its use with a healthcare provider, particularly for serious conditions, to ensure that it is appropriate and safe.

In conclusion, the basics of homeopathy are rooted in a philosophy of treating the whole person and utilizing natural substances in a highly diluted form to stimulate the body's healing processes. Its individualized, holistic approach to wellness continues to appeal to many seeking natural alternatives for health and healing. While it remains a topic of debate in scientific circles, its longstanding presence and the growing number of patients who seek its benefits underscore its continued relevance in the realm of alternative medicine.

Homeopathic Remedies

Homeopathic remedies are a cornerstone of homeopathic medicine, designed to stimulate the body's natural healing processes. These remedies are created by diluting natural substances—typically plants, minerals, or animal products—through a series of steps, each time shaking the mixture to enhance its healing properties. According to the principles of homeopathy, these highly diluted solutions carry the "energetic imprint" of the original substance, which is believed to help balance the body's vital force and restore health.

A key aspect of homeopathic remedies is their individualized approach. Practitioners assess a person's physical, mental, and emotional symptoms before prescribing a remedy, aiming to match the remedy to the person's unique set of characteristics rather than simply treating a disease. This personalized approach makes homeopathy distinct from conventional medicine, which typically focuses on diagnosing and treating specific illnesses.

Some of the most widely used homeopathic remedies have become well-known for their effectiveness in treating various common ailments. **Arnica montana**, derived from the mountain daisy, is one of the most popular remedies for trauma, bruising, and muscle soreness. It is often used to reduce pain, swelling, and inflammation following injuries, surgery, or intense physical activity. Many athletes and individuals recovering from injuries turn to arnica for its ability to speed up healing and alleviate discomfort.

Belladonna, derived from the deadly nightshade plant, is commonly used to treat conditions characterized by sudden, intense symptoms such as fever, inflammation, and throbbing pain. It is often prescribed for conditions like **tonsillitis**, **sinus infections**, and **earaches**, where symptoms appear rapidly and are accompanied by a high fever. The remedy is thought to help calm the body's reaction to inflammation and reduce fever, bringing about a more balanced state.

Another frequently used remedy is **Nux vomica**, made from the seeds of the strychnine tree. This remedy is often recommended for individuals experiencing **digestive issues**, such as indigestion, nausea, or constipation, especially when triggered by overindulgence in food, alcohol, or stress. It is also used to treat irritability, fatigue, and the effects of a sedentary lifestyle, making it useful for people dealing with the physical and mental toll of modern, fast-paced living.

Calendula, derived from the marigold flower, is known for its remarkable healing properties for the skin. It is commonly used to treat cuts, scrapes, burns, and other superficial wounds. Calendula is believed to promote tissue regeneration, prevent infection, and soothe inflammation. Many people use it in the form of creams, gels, or tinctures to promote faster healing of minor injuries and to reduce scarring.

For **allergies** and **hay fever**, **Allium cepa** (red onion) is a common remedy. It is used to treat symptoms like watery eyes, sneezing, and a runny nose, which are characteristic of allergic rhinitis. Since the symptoms of hay fever are similar to those caused by cutting onions—such as tearing and nasal discharge—the use of Allium cepa is based on the homeopathic principle of "like cures like."

Rhus toxicodendron, made from poison ivy, is frequently used to treat **muscle and joint pain** associated with conditions like arthritis or sprains. It is typically prescribed for pain that is worse with initial movement but improves with continued motion or warmth. This remedy is often used when pain is accompanied by stiffness, swelling, and a feeling of being "rusty" or "creaky," especially after rest or in the morning.

Another well-known remedy is **Chamomilla**, derived from the chamomile plant, which is commonly used for **irritability**, especially in children. It is often prescribed for teething pain, colic, or conditions where the person exhibits extreme sensitivity to pain, agitation, or frustration. Chamomilla is believed to help soothe the nervous system and calm emotional reactions, making it useful for individuals who are easily upset or distressed by minor discomfort.

Hypericum perforatum, also known as St. John's Wort, is used in homeopathy to treat nerve pain, particularly following injuries to areas rich in nerves, such as the fingers, toes, or spine. It is thought to promote nerve regeneration and reduce the severity of pain following trauma or surgery. Homeopaths commonly recommend Hypericum for conditions like **sciatica**, **shingles**, or **nerve injuries**, where there is sharp, shooting pain.

One of the strengths of homeopathic remedies is their ability to address **mental and emotional health**. Remedies such as **Ignatia amara**, derived from the St. Ignatius bean, are used to treat symptoms of emotional stress, grief, and anxiety. It is particularly helpful for individuals who are experiencing mood swings or a sense of emotional overwhelm following loss, disappointment, or emotional shock. Similarly, **Lycopodium clavatum**, made from club moss, is often used for anxiety-related issues, especially when individuals experience a lack of confidence or self-doubt.

The use of homeopathic remedies, though widely practiced by those seeking alternative medicine, remains controversial in the scientific community. While many people report positive outcomes from using homeopathic treatments, particularly for minor conditions, critics argue that the highly diluted nature of homeopathic remedies makes them unlikely to contain any active molecules, suggesting that their effectiveness could be due to the placebo effect. Despite this, homeopathy continues to be embraced by millions worldwide, and its individualized approach remains a cornerstone of holistic healthcare.

In conclusion, homeopathic remedies offer a natural, personalized approach to health, utilizing highly diluted substances to stimulate the body's healing processes. From treating common ailments like bruising and allergies to managing chronic pain and emotional stress, these remedies have become an integral part of alternative medicine for many individuals seeking gentle, non-invasive treatment options. Although the scientific community remains divided on the mechanisms behind homeopathy, its longstanding use and popularity highlight its ongoing place in the world of alternative healthcare.

Criticisms and Controversies

Alternative medicine has long been a topic of debate, with its practices, philosophies, and efficacy often subject to both praise and criticism. While millions of people worldwide turn to alternative therapies for relief from a variety of conditions, these approaches have sparked significant controversy within the medical community. Critics often point to a lack of scientific evidence, safety concerns, and the risk of delaying conventional treatments as major reasons for their skepticism. However, advocates of alternative medicine argue that these practices offer valuable options for individuals seeking holistic care, and in some cases, they can be beneficial when used alongside traditional medicine.

One of the primary criticisms of alternative medicine is the **lack of scientific evidence** supporting many of its practices. While some alternative therapies, such as acupuncture, herbal medicine, and chiropractic care, have been studied extensively, much of the evidence remains inconclusive or inconsistent. Many of the studies conducted on alternative treatments have small sample sizes, poor methodologies, or fail to demonstrate statistically significant results. In cases where positive effects have been reported, critics argue that the benefits could be due to **placebo effects**—the psychological phenomenon where patients experience improvements in their symptoms simply because they believe the treatment will work, rather than any inherent therapeutic properties of the treatment itself.

Another significant point of contention is the issue of **safety**. While many alternative treatments are generally considered safe, some can carry risks, particularly when used improperly or in combination with conventional medications. For example, certain herbal remedies, such as **St. John's Wort**, can interfere with the effectiveness of prescription drugs, including antidepressants, birth control pills, and blood thinners. Ingesting unregulated or improperly prepared herbal supplements can lead to toxicity or adverse reactions, especially when patients self-prescribe without guidance from a qualified practitioner. The lack of regulation in some alternative medicine industries also raises concerns about the quality and consistency of products, leading to potential contamination or inaccurate labeling.

Some forms of alternative medicine also face criticism for **delaying conventional medical treatment**, especially in cases where individuals opt for these therapies in place of evidence-based care for serious conditions like cancer, heart disease, or diabetes. There have been instances where patients, in seeking alternative treatments, avoid seeking proper medical attention or delay diagnosis and treatment of life-threatening conditions. This can lead to worsened health outcomes, particularly when time-sensitive treatments, such as surgery or chemotherapy, are required. The high-profile cases of celebrities and well-known figures who have promoted alternative treatments for serious conditions without the guidance of medical professionals often fuel concerns about the potential harm of delaying conventional care.

A further point of criticism is the **financial cost** associated with some alternative therapies. Many of these treatments, such as homeopathy, chiropractic care, or long-term acupuncture sessions, are often not covered by insurance, leaving patients to pay out of pocket. The high costs of some therapies can create a barrier to access for those who may already be dealing with chronic conditions or financial difficulties. Furthermore, some alternative medicine practitioners may charge significant fees for treatments that have not been proven effective, raising concerns about potential exploitation of vulnerable individuals seeking hope for relief.

Despite these criticisms, alternative medicine continues to grow in popularity, with increasing numbers of individuals seeking treatments that focus on holistic care and addressing the underlying causes of illness, rather than just symptoms. Many proponents argue that alternative therapies, when used properly and in conjunction with conventional medicine, offer valuable benefits. For example, therapies like **meditation**, **yoga**, and **massage therapy** have been shown to reduce stress, improve mental health, and provide relief from chronic pain. These practices are often embraced as part of an integrated approach to health, with individuals using them alongside medical treatment to improve overall well-being.

Some forms of alternative medicine, particularly those that emphasize the **mind-body connection**, have also received attention for their role in **preventing illness** and **promoting general wellness**. Practices such as mindfulness meditation, acupuncture, and herbal remedies may help reduce stress, boost immunity, and improve quality of life, particularly for individuals with chronic conditions. In these cases, alternative therapies are often seen as a complement to conventional medicine, supporting the patient's overall health and quality of life.

Another potential benefit of alternative medicine is the **individualized approach** that many therapies offer. While conventional medicine often focuses on treating specific diseases or conditions, alternative therapies take a more holistic view, considering the physical, emotional, and psychological aspects of a person's health. This approach can resonate with individuals who feel that conventional medicine does not fully address their needs or concerns. It also allows patients to take a more active role in their health and treatment choices.

Despite the controversies, alternative medicine remains a prominent part of global healthcare systems. For many people, these treatments offer solutions that align with their values, lifestyle, or belief systems about health. While there are valid concerns about safety, efficacy, and the potential for exploitation, there is also a growing recognition that alternative therapies, when properly researched, regulated, and used in combination with conventional medicine, can be valuable tools for health and wellness.

In conclusion, the criticisms and controversies surrounding alternative medicine are multifaceted, ranging from concerns about scientific evidence to issues of safety and the risk of delaying conventional treatments. While these criticisms are valid, they also highlight the need for rigorous scientific research, proper regulation, and responsible practice within the field. For those who choose to explore alternative therapies, it is important to seek guidance from qualified practitioners and maintain open communication with healthcare providers to ensure a balanced and informed approach to health and healing.

Aromatherapy

Aromatherapy is a form of alternative medicine that involves the use of essential oils and plant extracts to promote physical, emotional, and mental well-being. The practice has been used for thousands of years, with roots in ancient civilizations such as Egypt, China, and Greece, where aromatic plants were believed to have therapeutic properties. Today, aromatherapy is a popular complementary therapy that harnesses the power of scents to influence mood, reduce stress, and support overall health.

The primary focus of aromatherapy is the use of **essential oils**, which are highly concentrated extracts obtained from various parts of plants, including flowers, leaves, stems, and roots. These oils capture the plant's natural fragrance and therapeutic compounds, which are thought to have medicinal effects. Common essential oils used in aromatherapy include **lavender**, **peppermint, eucalyptus, chamomile**, and **tea tree oil**. Each oil has its own unique properties and can be used for a variety of health benefits.

One of the most well-known benefits of aromatherapy is its ability to promote **relaxation** and reduce **stress**. **Lavender essential oil**, in particular, is widely regarded for its calming effects. Research has shown that inhaling lavender oil can help reduce anxiety, lower blood pressure, and promote relaxation, making it a popular choice for people dealing with stress, insomnia, or even symptoms of depression. Studies have found that the scent of lavender can influence the limbic system of the brain, the part that controls emotions, helping to calm the nervous system.

Aromatherapy is also commonly used to treat **headaches** and **migraines**. **Peppermint oil** is often applied topically to the temples or inhaled for relief from tension headaches. The menthol in peppermint oil helps to relax muscles and improve circulation, providing a cooling sensation that can ease pain. Similarly, **eucalyptus oil**, with its strong menthol scent, is used to relieve sinus pressure and headaches associated with colds or allergies. The inhalation of these oils may help open up nasal passages, reduce congestion, and ease pain.

In addition to its effects on mood and relaxation, aromatherapy is also used for its **antimicrobial properties**. Essential oils like **tea tree oil** and **eucalyptus oil** are known for their ability to fight bacteria, viruses, and fungi. Tea tree oil, in particular, is commonly used in skincare products due to its ability to treat acne, soothe skin irritations, and promote wound healing. It has natural antiseptic and antifungal properties, making it effective in treating minor cuts, burns, and fungal infections like athlete's foot.

For those seeking natural ways to improve their **sleep**, aromatherapy offers several options. **Lavender oil** is again a popular choice, as its sedative effects help calm the mind and promote restful sleep. A study published in the *Journal of Sleep Research* found that lavender aroma could improve sleep quality, especially in individuals suffering from mild insomnia. Other essential oils, such as **chamomile** and **bergamot**, are also used in aromatherapy to alleviate insomnia and improve sleep patterns by soothing the nervous system.

Aromatherapy can also be beneficial in **enhancing focus** and cognitive performance. **Peppermint** and **rosemary oils** are commonly used to stimulate mental clarity and concentration.

Studies have shown that the aroma of peppermint can improve alertness, cognitive performance, and memory. Similarly, rosemary has been linked to improved concentration and mental performance, making it an ideal oil for students or those needing a mental boost during long hours of work.

While the therapeutic benefits of aromatherapy are widely acknowledged, it is essential to use essential oils safely. Due to their concentrated nature, essential oils should always be diluted before applying to the skin to avoid irritation or allergic reactions. Some oils, such as peppermint and eucalyptus, should be avoided by individuals with certain medical conditions, such as respiratory disorders or skin sensitivities. Pregnant women and young children should also exercise caution when using essential oils, as certain oils can have adverse effects during pregnancy or on developing children.

One of the simplest ways to use aromatherapy is through **diffusers**, which disperse essential oils into the air. This method allows the oil's scent to fill the room, providing a calming or invigorating atmosphere, depending on the oil used. **Topical application** is another popular method, where oils are diluted with a carrier oil (such as coconut or jojoba oil) and applied to the skin. Inhaling the scent directly from a bottle or adding a few drops of oil to a warm bath are also effective ways to experience the benefits of aromatherapy.

In conclusion, aromatherapy offers a natural and effective way to promote emotional, mental, and physical well-being. By harnessing the therapeutic properties of essential oils, aromatherapy can help reduce stress, alleviate pain, improve sleep, and support overall health. Whether used to enhance mood, boost cognitive function, or treat common ailments, aromatherapy remains a valuable tool in the realm of alternative medicine. When used safely and appropriately, it provides a holistic approach to health that complements traditional treatments and supports overall wellness.

Understanding Aromatherapy

Aromatherapy is a therapeutic practice that uses essential oils extracted from plants to enhance well-being and support health. It has been used for centuries, drawing on the natural healing properties of plant-based substances to treat a variety of physical, emotional, and mental conditions. Aromatherapy works by stimulating the sense of smell, which directly impacts the brain's limbic system—the area responsible for emotions, memory, and behavior—helping to create a sense of balance and relaxation.

Essential oils, the cornerstone of aromatherapy, are concentrated liquids derived from different parts of plants, including flowers, leaves, bark, roots, and fruit. These oils are highly potent and are thought to contain the plant's natural healing compounds, which can have various effects on the body. For example, **lavender** oil is known for its calming and relaxing properties, while **peppermint** oil is often used to invigorate the mind and relieve physical discomfort, such as headaches or muscle pain.

One of the primary ways aromatherapy works is by inhaling the aromas of these oils. The molecules from essential oils are absorbed into the olfactory system through the nose, which sends signals to the limbic system of the brain. This interaction can trigger the release of chemicals like endorphins, which help regulate mood and reduce stress. For example, **chamomile** and

lavender oils are often used to promote relaxation, helping to reduce anxiety and improve sleep quality. The calming effects of these oils make them a popular choice for individuals struggling with insomnia or high levels of stress.

In addition to emotional benefits, aromatherapy has been found to have several **physical health benefits**. **Peppermint** oil, with its cooling properties, is widely used to relieve symptoms of tension headaches, sinus congestion, and digestive issues. Its menthol content can help open up the airways, improve circulation, and promote digestion, making it a versatile and widely used oil in therapeutic settings. Similarly, **eucalyptus oil** is known for its antimicrobial and anti-inflammatory properties, often used to treat respiratory issues like colds, coughs, or congestion.

Aromatherapy can also be an effective treatment for **pain relief**. **Ginger** and **turmeric** essential oils, both known for their anti-inflammatory properties, can help reduce joint pain and muscle stiffness associated with conditions like arthritis. When applied topically (with proper dilution) or inhaled, these oils may work to soothe sore muscles and reduce swelling. Many people turn to these oils as a natural alternative to traditional painkillers, especially for chronic pain conditions.

One of the most common methods of using aromatherapy is through a **diffuser**, a device that disperses essential oils into the air, allowing the beneficial properties of the oils to be inhaled throughout the room. This method is ideal for improving mood, creating a calming environment, or purifying the air. **Topical application** of essential oils is also common, where oils are diluted with a carrier oil, such as coconut or jojoba oil, and massaged into the skin. This method is effective for treating localized pain, inflammation, or skin conditions like acne and eczema. **Baths** with a few drops of essential oil added to the water can provide a relaxing and therapeutic experience as the skin absorbs the oils.

In addition to these more common methods, aromatherapy can be integrated into everyday activities. For example, applying a few drops of **peppermint** oil to the temples or the back of the neck may help alleviate headache symptoms. Similarly, **frankincense oil** has been traditionally used in meditation practices to promote mental clarity, calm the mind, and enhance spiritual well-being.

While aromatherapy is generally safe when used correctly, it is important to follow safety guidelines, especially since essential oils are highly concentrated. Certain oils, such as **oregano** and **thyme**, can be irritating to the skin and should always be diluted before topical application. Pregnant women, individuals with certain medical conditions, and young children should exercise caution when using aromatherapy, as some oils may not be suitable for their health needs.

One of the appealing aspects of aromatherapy is its ability to work alongside other **alternative** or **conventional treatments**. When used in combination with other wellness practices, such as **yoga**, **massage therapy**, or **mindfulness meditation**, aromatherapy can enhance overall well-being and provide additional support for stress management, physical healing, and emotional balance.

In conclusion, aromatherapy is a holistic therapy that utilizes the power of essential oils to improve health and well-being. Its wide-ranging benefits, from relaxation and stress reduction to physical pain relief and immune support, make it a popular and versatile form of alternative medicine. By understanding the properties of various essential oils and how they interact with the body, individuals can harness the power of aromatherapy to support their overall health and enhance their quality of life.

Benefits and Uses

Alternative medicine offers a wide range of therapies and treatments that focus on promoting healing, preventing illness, and improving overall well-being without relying solely on conventional pharmaceutical approaches. These practices often prioritize the body's ability to heal itself, using natural remedies and holistic methods. The benefits and uses of alternative medicine are diverse, encompassing everything from physical health improvements to emotional and mental wellness.

One of the most well-known benefits of alternative medicine is its ability to address **chronic pain** and **musculoskeletal conditions**. Therapies like **acupuncture, chiropractic care**, and **massage therapy** are widely used to treat back pain, arthritis, migraines, and muscle tension. Acupuncture, for instance, involves the insertion of thin needles at specific points on the body, which can help alleviate pain by stimulating the body's natural pain-relief mechanisms and improving circulation. Chiropractic care, focusing on spinal adjustments, has been shown to provide relief from neck and back pain, as well as headaches. Massage therapy, with its ability to relax muscles and improve blood flow, is commonly used to treat conditions like fibromyalgia, tension headaches, and sports injuries.

Herbal medicine is another significant form of alternative treatment with wide-ranging benefits. Many herbs, such as **echinacea, ginger**, and **turmeric**, have demonstrated medicinal properties and are used to support the immune system, reduce inflammation, and treat digestive disorders. For example, **ginger** is often used to relieve nausea and digestive upset, while **turmeric**, with its active compound curcumin, is known for its powerful anti-inflammatory effects. Herbal remedies, often used in combination with other treatments, can help prevent illness, support recovery from illness, and promote general health.

Mental health is also an area where alternative medicine has found significant applications. Practices such as **yoga**, **meditation**, and **aromatherapy** have proven effective in reducing **stress**, improving **mood**, and treating conditions like **anxiety** and **depression**. Yoga and meditation work by focusing on mindfulness, improving body awareness, and calming the mind. These practices have been linked to lower levels of cortisol (the stress hormone) and increased production of **endorphins**, which promote feelings of happiness and well-being. **Aromatherapy**, which uses essential oils like **lavender** and **chamomile**, is commonly used to promote relaxation and improve sleep. Lavender oil, in particular, has been shown in studies to reduce anxiety and promote restful sleep, making it a popular remedy for those with insomnia or stress-related conditions.

Another key benefit of alternative medicine is its emphasis on **prevention** and **wellness**. Practices like **nutritional counseling**, **detoxification**, and **herbal supplements** aim to support the body's natural processes and prevent the onset of illness. Nutritional approaches, such as dietary adjustments or supplementation with **vitamins** and **minerals**, help individuals maintain optimal health and boost immunity. Detoxification programs, which can include herbal cleanses or fasting under professional guidance, aim to remove toxins from the body, improving overall health and energy levels.

Holistic therapies, such as **homeopathy** and **energy healing**, focus on treating the individual as a whole, addressing not just the symptoms but also the root causes of illness. Homeopathy, for example, involves using highly diluted substances to stimulate the body's healing responses. Advocates of this therapy believe it can help balance emotional, mental, and physical health. **Reiki** and other forms of **energy healing** work on the premise that the body's energy can be manipulated to promote healing and restore balance. These treatments are often used to help manage stress, reduce pain, and support emotional healing.

In addition to treating specific conditions, alternative medicine is often used to improve **overall quality of life**. Many people turn to therapies like **acupuncture**, **yoga**, or **massage** not just for pain relief, but to enhance their overall health, improve their flexibility, increase energy levels, and promote relaxation. These treatments can support the body's natural systems, encourage a sense of balance, and contribute to long-term wellness by addressing both physical and emotional needs.

Aromatherapy and **herbal medicine** also play a significant role in **immunity support**. For example, **echinacea** and **elderberry** have long been used to support immune function, helping the body fend off infections, particularly during cold and flu season. Similarly, **garlic**, known for its antimicrobial properties, has been used as a natural remedy to fight infections and strengthen the immune system.

For individuals seeking natural alternatives to conventional medications, **alternative medicine** offers a range of safe and effective options. Whether used for **pain management, stress reduction, immune support**, or general wellness, these therapies provide a holistic approach to health that emphasizes balance, prevention, and the body's intrinsic ability to heal itself.

While the efficacy of some alternative treatments is still under research and debate, many individuals report significant improvements in their health and well-being through their use. As a complementary approach to conventional medicine, alternative therapies can support a healthier lifestyle and provide relief from a variety of physical and emotional challenges. However, it is always important to consult with healthcare providers before embarking on alternative treatments, particularly for serious or chronic conditions.

Essential Oils Guide

Essential oils are concentrated plant extracts that have been used for centuries in aromatherapy, skincare, and medicinal practices. Derived from various parts of plants—such as flowers, leaves, bark, stems, and roots—these oils contain the natural compounds that give plants their distinctive scents and therapeutic properties. In alternative medicine, essential oils are often used to promote physical, emotional, and mental well-being. When used correctly, they can support a range of health benefits, from stress relief and pain management to improving skin health and supporting the immune system.

One of the most popular uses of essential oils is for **stress relief** and **relaxation**. **Lavender oil** is perhaps the most widely known for its calming effects, frequently used to reduce anxiety, promote restful sleep, and calm the nervous system. Lavender oil can be inhaled through a diffuser or applied topically (diluted in a carrier oil) to relieve tension and anxiety. **Chamomile** and **bergamot** oils are also commonly used for their ability to calm the mind, reduce emotional tension, and support mental clarity.

Essential oils can also be incredibly effective for managing **pain** and **inflammation**. **Peppermint oil**, for example, contains menthol, which has a cooling effect and is often used to relieve headaches, muscle pain, and tension. Applied to the temples or neck, peppermint oil can provide quick relief from tension headaches. Similarly, **eucalyptus oil** is known for its anti-inflammatory properties and is often used for sore muscles and joint pain. It is particularly useful when combined with a carrier oil for a soothing massage or added to a warm bath to relax stiff muscles.

For individuals suffering from **digestive issues**, essential oils offer natural relief as well. **Ginger** oil is widely recognized for its ability to alleviate nausea, improve digestion, and reduce bloating. Whether you're dealing with morning sickness, motion sickness, or general digestive discomfort, ginger essential oil can be inhaled or applied topically on the abdomen to help soothe digestive upset. **Peppermint oil** also plays a role in digestive health, as it can help relax the muscles of the gastrointestinal tract, reducing symptoms of irritable bowel syndrome (IBS), indigestion, and gas.

Essential oils are also commonly used for **skin health**. Many oils have antimicrobial, anti-inflammatory, and antioxidant properties that can help heal and protect the skin. **Tea tree oil**, for example, is well-known for its antibacterial and antifungal properties, making it a go-to remedy for acne, fungal infections, and minor cuts. **Frankincense oil** has anti-aging properties and is often used to improve skin tone, reduce the appearance of wrinkles, and promote the regeneration of skin cells. It is frequently added to skincare routines for its rejuvenating effects.

In addition to skincare, essential oils can be incredibly beneficial for **immune support**. Oils like **lemon, eucalyptus**, and **tea tree** are known for their ability to purify the air and support respiratory health. They have natural antiviral, antibacterial, and antifungal properties that help protect the body from infections. **Lemon oil** is particularly effective for boosting immunity, as its high vitamin C content helps strengthen the body's defense mechanisms. **Thieves oil**, a blend of clove, lemon, cinnamon, eucalyptus, and rosemary, is also popular for its powerful antimicrobial properties and is commonly used to combat colds and flu.

Aromatherapy is a primary way in which essential oils are used to affect mood and emotional health. Simply inhaling certain scents can have a profound impact on mood and stress levels. **Citrus oils**, such as **orange**, **lemon**, and **grapefruit**, are often used for their uplifting and energizing effects. These oils are commonly used in the morning to boost mood, improve mental clarity, and increase energy levels. **Ylang-ylang**, **sandalwood**, and **rose** oils, on the other hand, have calming and grounding effects, making them ideal for reducing stress and fostering a sense of emotional balance.

When using essential oils, it's essential to follow safety guidelines. **Dilution** is crucial because pure essential oils are highly concentrated and can cause skin irritation or adverse reactions if applied directly. They should always be mixed with a **carrier oil** such as **coconut oil**, **jojoba oil**, or **almond oil** for safe topical application. Essential oils should also be used with caution around children, pregnant women, and individuals with specific health conditions, as some oils may not be suitable for these groups.

Inhalation is another common method for using essential oils, either through **diffusers**, steam inhalation, or simply adding a few drops to a tissue or cotton ball. A diffuser is a great way to disperse essential oils into the air, allowing their aromatic properties to fill a room and promote a calming or invigorating environment. When using oils for inhalation, be sure to use them in well-ventilated areas and avoid prolonged exposure to strong scents, especially in closed spaces.

Bathing with essential oils is another effective way to experience their therapeutic effects. Adding a few drops of essential oil to a warm bath can help relax the body, ease muscle tension, and promote a sense of calm. For a more relaxing experience, oils like **lavender, chamomile,** and **sandalwood** are ideal, while oils like **peppermint** and **citrus** can help revitalize and energize the body.

In conclusion, essential oils are a powerful tool in alternative medicine, offering a wide range of therapeutic benefits. Whether used for **pain relief, stress reduction, skin health,** or **immune support**, essential oils can provide natural and effective solutions to common health concerns. By understanding how different oils work and using them safely, individuals can integrate aromatherapy into their wellness routines for enhanced physical and emotional well-being.

Chiropractic Medicine

Chiropractic medicine is a form of alternative therapy that focuses on diagnosing and treating musculoskeletal disorders, particularly those related to the spine. The core philosophy of chiropractic care is that the body's structure—especially the spine—plays a critical role in overall health, and that misalignments in the spine, called **subluxations**, can interfere with the body's nervous system and lead to a variety of health issues. Chiropractors use hands-on spinal manipulation and other techniques to help align the body's musculoskeletal structure, thereby improving function and relieving pain.

The **spinal adjustment** is the primary treatment method used in chiropractic care. During an adjustment, chiropractors use controlled, sudden force applied to specific joints in the spine or other parts of the body to restore proper alignment. This can help alleviate pressure on the nervous system, improve circulation, and enhance the body's natural healing processes. While spinal adjustments are the most commonly used technique, chiropractors may also employ other methods, such as massage, exercise, heat or cold therapy, and nutritional counseling to address a wide range of health concerns.

One of the most well-known and widely practiced benefits of chiropractic care is its effectiveness in treating **back pain**, **neck pain**, and **headaches**. Numerous studies have shown that chiropractic adjustments can provide significant relief for individuals suffering from chronic back pain, especially when combined with other therapies like physical therapy or lifestyle changes. Chiropractic care has been found to be particularly effective for lower back pain, with research indicating that spinal manipulation can help reduce pain, improve mobility, and prevent recurrence. Similarly, many people turn to chiropractic treatments for tension headaches or migraines, as spinal adjustments can help reduce the frequency and intensity of these debilitating conditions by releasing tension in the neck and shoulders.

Beyond pain management, chiropractic care is also used to promote overall **wellness** and **preventative health**. Chiropractors believe that maintaining proper alignment of the spine can improve the body's ability to function optimally. By ensuring that the nervous system is not compromised by spinal misalignments, chiropractic care aims to improve immune system function, enhance energy levels, and boost the body's natural ability to heal itself. Regular chiropractic check-ups are often recommended to prevent future health issues and to support long-term wellness.

Sports injuries are another area where chiropractic care has gained popularity. Chiropractors work with athletes to treat and prevent musculoskeletal injuries, including strains, sprains, and joint injuries. Spinal adjustments, along with other manual therapies, can help restore range of motion, reduce inflammation, and speed up recovery time. Chiropractic care is often used in combination with other sports medicine treatments to help athletes recover from injuries and improve their performance.

In addition to physical health, chiropractic medicine also emphasizes the mind-body connection. Chiropractors believe that by improving spinal alignment, they can help address emotional and psychological issues that may arise from physical discomfort or misalignments. For example, some patients report that chiropractic adjustments help improve their mood, reduce feelings of stress, and promote better sleep. This holistic approach to treatment considers the interconnectedness of the body's systems and aims to treat not only the symptoms but the root causes of illness or discomfort.

Chiropractic medicine has faced its share of skepticism and controversy, particularly regarding its **effectiveness** for conditions that are not musculoskeletal in nature. While many studies support chiropractic care for managing back pain, there is less consensus regarding its ability to treat conditions such as asthma, allergies, or digestive issues. Some critics argue that chiropractic treatments should be reserved for musculoskeletal concerns and that the broader claims of chiropractic care lack scientific backing. However, advocates of chiropractic medicine emphasize the importance of a **holistic** approach to health and argue that spinal health plays a critical role in the proper functioning of the body as a whole.

As with any form of healthcare, chiropractic treatment has potential **risks**. While spinal manipulation is generally safe, there is a small risk of injury, such as muscle strains or, in rare cases, more serious complications like a herniated disc or stroke, especially when performed incorrectly. It is essential to seek care from a licensed chiropractor who has received proper training and adheres to established safety protocols. Additionally, individuals with certain medical conditions, such as severe osteoporosis, fractures, or spinal tumors, may need to avoid chiropractic treatments or consult with a healthcare provider before seeking chiropractic care.

Chiropractic care is generally considered safe and effective for many people, especially for those dealing with musculoskeletal pain. It is often used as a complementary treatment alongside conventional medical therapies. Many people who experience chronic pain or discomfort turn to chiropractors when traditional medical treatments, such as medication or surgery, have not provided adequate relief. Chiropractors often work alongside other healthcare providers to ensure a holistic, patient-centered approach to care.

In conclusion, chiropractic medicine offers a non-invasive, drug-free treatment option for managing pain, promoting overall wellness, and addressing musculoskeletal issues. Through spinal adjustments and other therapeutic techniques, chiropractic care can help restore balance to the body, improve function, and relieve discomfort. Whether used for managing back pain, enhancing athletic performance, or supporting long-term health, chiropractic care remains a popular and widely respected form of alternative medicine.

An Introduction to Chiropractic Medicine

Chiropractic medicine is a form of alternative therapy that focuses on diagnosing and treating musculoskeletal disorders, particularly those related to the spine. The core belief behind chiropractic care is that the alignment of the spine plays a central role in overall health. According to chiropractic philosophy, misalignments in the spine, known as **subluxations**, can interfere with the nervous system, leading to pain, dysfunction, and a range of health issues. Chiropractors use hands-on spinal manipulation and other techniques to restore proper alignment, improve bodily function, and alleviate pain.

The practice of chiropractic medicine is built around the concept that the body is capable of healing itself, particularly when the nervous system is functioning optimally. Chiropractors believe that by adjusting the spine and other joints, they can remove barriers to the body's innate ability to maintain health. The most common technique used in chiropractic care is spinal manipulation, also known as **spinal adjustments**, which involves applying controlled pressure to specific joints in the spine or other areas of the body to correct misalignments.

Chiropractic care is widely known for its effectiveness in treating **back pain**, **neck pain**, and **headaches**, with a strong focus on conditions related to the spine. It has gained popularity as a non-invasive, drug-free alternative to traditional treatments. Many individuals with chronic back pain or other musculoskeletal issues turn to chiropractors for relief when other methods, such as medication or surgery, have proven ineffective. Chiropractors are trained to assess and treat musculoskeletal issues, using a variety of techniques to relieve pain and improve mobility.

Beyond pain management, chiropractic care is also used to promote **overall wellness**. Many chiropractors recommend regular adjustments to maintain spinal health, prevent injury, and improve the body's ability to function at its best. Some patients seek chiropractic care for general health and prevention, as it is believed to improve immune function, energy levels, and posture. Chiropractic care is often used in conjunction with other health practices, such as physical therapy, massage, or exercise, to support overall physical well-being.

While spinal manipulation is the primary treatment used in chiropractic care, chiropractors may also use other complementary therapies to address a variety of conditions. These can include **soft tissue therapies** like massage or stretching, **nutritional counseling**, **posture correction**, and **exercise recommendations** to improve strength and flexibility. Chiropractors take a holistic approach, considering the entire body and its functions, and often educate patients about healthy lifestyle habits to prevent future health issues.

Chiropractic medicine has its roots in the late 19th century, when **Daniel David Palmer**, a Canadian-born healer, founded the profession. Palmer believed that the spine's alignment was integral to health, and he performed the first spinal adjustment on a patient in 1895. His work paved the way for chiropractic medicine to evolve into a recognized form of healthcare that is now practiced worldwide.

Although chiropractic care is widely respected and used, it has faced its share of controversy and skepticism. Critics have questioned the scientific validity of certain chiropractic practices, particularly when it comes to claims of treating conditions that are not directly related to the spine, such as asthma or digestive disorders. Some individuals remain cautious of chiropractic adjustments due to concerns over the safety of spinal manipulation, particularly in vulnerable populations. However, numerous studies support the effectiveness of chiropractic care, particularly for musculoskeletal issues like back and neck pain. Many health organizations, including the World Health Organization (WHO), recognize chiropractic care as a legitimate treatment option for specific conditions.

In conclusion, chiropractic medicine offers a non-invasive, drug-free approach to treating musculoskeletal disorders, with a focus on spinal health and overall wellness. By using spinal adjustments and other complementary techniques, chiropractors aim to improve the functioning of the nervous system, relieve pain, and promote the body's natural healing abilities. Whether used for managing chronic pain or for maintaining overall health, chiropractic care continues to be a popular choice for individuals seeking alternative, holistic treatment options.

Pros and Cons

Alternative medicine offers a broad range of therapies and practices designed to promote health and well-being without relying on conventional pharmaceuticals or surgeries. Many people turn to alternative medicine for its holistic approach, aiming to treat the root causes of ailments rather than just symptoms. However, like any form of treatment, it comes with both benefits and drawbacks. Understanding the pros and cons of alternative medicine can help individuals make informed choices about their healthcare options.

Pros of Alternative Medicine

1. **Holistic Approach to Health**: One of the key advantages of alternative medicine is its emphasis on treating the whole person, rather than just targeting specific symptoms or diseases. Many alternative therapies, such as acupuncture, naturopathy, and homeopathy, consider physical, emotional, and spiritual health, aiming to restore balance and promote overall wellness.
2. **Natural Remedies**: Many alternative treatments use natural substances, such as herbs, essential oils, and plant-based compounds, which some individuals prefer over synthetic medications. These natural remedies often appeal to those seeking less invasive, chemical-free solutions to their health problems.
3. **Fewer Side Effects**: When used correctly, alternative therapies like herbal medicine, acupuncture, and

massage therapy tend to have fewer and less severe side effects than conventional pharmaceuticals. This is particularly appealing for individuals who experience adverse reactions to prescription medications or who prefer to avoid pharmaceutical interventions.
4. **Personalized Care**: Alternative medicine often involves a more personalized approach to healthcare. Practitioners typically spend more time getting to know their patients, including their lifestyle, emotional state, and personal health history, which allows them to tailor treatments to the individual's specific needs.
5. **Focus on Prevention**: Many alternative medicine practices emphasize **prevention** rather than just treatment. Techniques such as nutritional counseling, stress management, and exercise recommendations aim to prevent illness and improve long-term health, rather than just addressing immediate symptoms or conditions.
6. **Complementary to Conventional Medicine**: Alternative medicine can often be used alongside conventional treatments to enhance their effectiveness. For example, acupuncture or massage therapy may complement physical therapy in the treatment of musculoskeletal pain, or aromatherapy may be used to reduce stress during cancer treatment.

Cons of Alternative Medicine

1. **Lack of Scientific Evidence**: One of the main criticisms of alternative medicine is the lack of rigorous scientific research to support the efficacy of many treatments. While some therapies, like acupuncture and chiropractic care, have been studied extensively, others, such as homeopathy, remain controversial due to insufficient clinical evidence proving their effectiveness.
2. **Risk of Delaying Conventional Treatment**: Some individuals may turn to alternative medicine exclusively,

foregoing conventional medical treatments for serious conditions like cancer, heart disease, or diabetes. In such cases, relying solely on alternative therapies can delay diagnosis and treatment, potentially leading to worsened health outcomes.
3. **Unregulated Practices**: In many areas, the alternative medicine industry is not as strictly regulated as conventional medicine. This lack of oversight can lead to varying quality and safety standards, with some practitioners lacking formal training or offering treatments that may be ineffective or even harmful. This can be particularly concerning with herbal supplements, which may be contaminated or improperly labeled.
4. **Potential for Harmful Interactions**: Some alternative treatments, particularly herbal supplements, can interact negatively with prescription medications, leading to unwanted side effects or reduced effectiveness of conventional treatments. For example, **St. John's Wort** can interfere with antidepressants and birth control pills, while **garlic** in large doses can thin the blood and increase the risk of bleeding when combined with blood thinners.
5. **Cost**: Alternative medicine treatments are often not covered by insurance, meaning individuals may need to pay out-of-pocket for therapies like acupuncture, chiropractic care, or naturopathic consultations. Additionally, some alternative treatments can be costly over the long term, especially if regular sessions or ongoing treatments are required.
6. **Placebo Effect**: Some critics argue that many alternative medicine therapies are effective primarily due to the placebo effect—the psychological phenomenon where patients experience improvement simply because they believe a treatment will work. While the placebo effect can still have real benefits, relying on it without

addressing the root cause of a health issue may limit long-term results.

In conclusion, alternative medicine offers a range of benefits, from a holistic approach to health and natural remedies to personalized care and a focus on prevention. However, it also carries risks, including a lack of scientific backing for certain treatments, potential delays in conventional medical care, and unregulated practices. It is important for individuals to weigh these pros and cons, consult with healthcare professionals, and make informed decisions when considering alternative medicine as part of their overall health and wellness plan.

Chiropractic Techniques

Chiropractic techniques are focused on diagnosing and treating musculoskeletal disorders, particularly those related to the spine, using hands-on methods to restore proper alignment and function. Chiropractors believe that misalignments in the spine, known as **subluxations**, can interfere with the body's nervous system and lead to a wide range of health problems. By applying specific spinal adjustments and other manual therapies, chiropractors aim to promote healing, alleviate pain, and improve overall health.

Spinal Manipulation (Spinal Adjustments) is the most well-known chiropractic technique. During this procedure, chiropractors apply a controlled, sudden force to a joint in the spine, typically using their hands or specialized instruments. The goal is to correct misalignments and improve spinal motion. Spinal manipulation is particularly effective in treating conditions such as lower back pain, neck pain, headaches, and certain types of musculoskeletal discomfort. Research has shown that spinal adjustments can provide significant relief for many people suffering from chronic pain, especially in the lower back and neck.

Activator Method is another chiropractic technique that uses a small, handheld device called the **Activator Adjusting Instrument**. This device delivers a gentle impulse to specific points on the spine, which is intended to restore proper alignment without the need for manual force or sudden thrusts. The Activator Method is often used for patients who may have sensitive joints, are older, or prefer a less forceful treatment. It is effective for treating various conditions, including joint dysfunctions, headaches, and spinal misalignments.

Diversified Technique is one of the most common methods used by chiropractors. It involves a combination of high-velocity, low-amplitude adjustments aimed at improving spinal motion and realigning misaligned vertebrae. The practitioner uses their hands to apply force directly to specific spinal joints, often with a quick thrust that may produce a popping sound, which is the release of gas from the joints. The Diversified Technique is used to treat a variety of musculoskeletal conditions, including back pain, neck pain, and sciatica, by addressing spinal misalignments and improving the function of the nervous system.

Thompson Technique involves the use of a specialized table with sections that drop when pressure is applied. The chiropractor adjusts the position of the patient and applies gentle pressure to the spine. As the chiropractor applies force, the table "drops," allowing for a more comfortable adjustment that reduces the amount of force required. This technique is particularly useful for people with conditions like **sciatica** or those who may experience discomfort from other adjustment techniques. It is effective in realigning the spine and reducing pain while minimizing strain on the body.

Gonstead Technique is a highly specific chiropractic technique that focuses on assessing and correcting spinal misalignments through detailed analysis and adjustments. Chiropractors trained in this technique use a combination of visual analysis, palpation (feeling the spine), and X-rays to determine the precise area of misalignment. The goal of the Gonstead Technique is to correct spinal dysfunction and improve nervous system function, leading to pain relief and improved mobility. This technique is often used for patients with chronic back pain, sciatica, or herniated discs.

Flexion-Distraction Technique is a non-force, hands-on approach used primarily for disc issues, including **herniated or bulging discs**. This technique involves the use of a specialized table that gently stretches and flexes the spine. By gently pulling and decompressing the spine, the flexion-distraction technique reduces pressure on the spinal discs and nerve roots, helping to alleviate pain and improve mobility. It is particularly effective for conditions like **lumbar disc herniations**, **sciatica**, and other disc-related issues.

Soft Tissue Therapy is often incorporated into chiropractic care to address muscle stiffness and tightness that can contribute to pain and discomfort. Chiropractors may use techniques such as **massage**, **trigger point therapy**, and **myofascial release** to help relax muscles, improve circulation, and reduce inflammation. Soft tissue therapies can enhance the effectiveness of spinal adjustments and are frequently used in conjunction with other chiropractic treatments to provide holistic care.

Kinesiology is a technique that involves muscle testing to identify imbalances or weaknesses in the body. Chiropractors who use this approach assess the strength and function of various muscles in relation to specific spinal segments. By detecting abnormal muscle responses, the chiropractor can determine the underlying causes of discomfort or dysfunction and adjust the spine or recommend exercises to improve muscle strength and coordination. Kinesiology is particularly useful for diagnosing issues related to the nervous system and muscular-skeletal health.

Postural Restoration Therapy (PRT) focuses on the alignment and restoration of normal posture to prevent pain and improve function. Chiropractors using this method analyze the posture and movement patterns of their patients and design customized exercises to address any postural imbalances. Poor posture can contribute to a wide range of musculoskeletal issues, including back and neck pain, headaches, and joint problems, making PRT an important aspect of preventive chiropractic care.

In conclusion, chiropractic techniques offer a variety of methods aimed at improving spinal health, alleviating pain, and promoting overall well-being. Whether through spinal adjustments, non-invasive therapies, or specialized techniques like the Activator Method or Flexion-Distraction, chiropractic care provides a versatile, holistic approach to musculoskeletal health. These techniques are designed not only to treat pain but to enhance the body's ability to heal itself, restore function, and improve quality of life. By using a combination of hands-on techniques and therapeutic approaches, chiropractors can help patients achieve better health and mobility.

Nutrition and Diet Therapy

Nutrition and diet therapy in alternative medicine focuses on the relationship between what we eat and how it affects our overall health. This approach emphasizes the healing power of food and its role in preventing, managing, and even reversing certain health conditions. Unlike conventional medicine, which often relies on pharmaceuticals to treat symptoms, nutrition and diet therapy seek to address the root causes of ailments by modifying eating habits and incorporating nutrient-dense foods into daily life.

One of the primary principles of diet therapy is the idea that food can serve as medicine. By consuming a variety of nutrient-rich foods, individuals can support the body's natural healing processes, boost immunity, and improve overall well-being. Specific dietary adjustments are made to target certain health conditions, improve energy levels, and promote mental clarity. For instance, **anti-inflammatory diets** are often recommended for people with chronic conditions like arthritis, where the goal is to reduce inflammation through the inclusion of foods that have natural anti-inflammatory properties.

For individuals dealing with **chronic diseases** such as **diabetes**, **heart disease**, or **high blood pressure**, nutrition and diet therapy can play a crucial role in managing these conditions. Diets that are rich in fiber, low in processed sugars, and high in heart-healthy fats, such as the **Mediterranean diet**, are commonly recommended. This type of diet focuses on fresh fruits, vegetables, whole grains, lean proteins, and healthy fats like olive oil, which have been shown to reduce the risk of cardiovascular issues and support overall metabolic health.

Detoxification diets are another popular approach in alternative medicine, aimed at eliminating toxins from the body and improving digestive health. These diets often include a combination of **juices, smoothies,** and **whole foods** that are high in antioxidants and fiber, with the goal of supporting the liver and kidneys, the body's primary detoxifying organs. Foods like **garlic, lemon,** and **green leafy vegetables** are frequently emphasized for their detoxifying properties. Proponents believe that by cleansing the body of accumulated toxins, people can experience increased energy, better digestion, and enhanced skin health.

For those suffering from **digestive disorders** like **irritable bowel syndrome (IBS)** or **food intolerances**, nutrition and diet therapy can provide significant relief. Personalized diets that eliminate or reduce trigger foods, such as dairy, gluten, or certain carbohydrates, can help ease symptoms and promote gut health. A **low FODMAP diet**, for example, is often recommended for individuals with IBS. This diet limits foods that are poorly absorbed in the small intestine, helping to reduce symptoms like bloating, gas, and abdominal pain.

Nutrition and diet therapy also recognizes the **mind-body connection** and its impact on emotional and psychological well-being. Diets that include foods rich in **omega-3 fatty acids**, **B vitamins**, and **antioxidants** have been shown to improve mental clarity and reduce symptoms of anxiety and depression. For example, foods like **fatty fish** (salmon, mackerel), **walnuts, flaxseeds,** and **leafy greens** are recommended for their brain-boosting properties. In addition, **fermented foods** like **yogurt, kimchi,** and **sauerkraut** support gut health by providing probiotics, which may play a role in reducing anxiety and improving mood through the gut-brain axis.

Another area where nutrition and diet therapy plays a key role is in **weight management** and **metabolism**. A balanced diet that emphasizes whole, unprocessed foods and avoids refined sugars, trans fats, and artificial additives is central to maintaining a healthy weight. Diets rich in fiber, such as those containing plenty of vegetables, fruits, legumes, and whole grains, can improve digestion, reduce hunger cravings, and support long-term weight loss goals. Additionally, adequate **hydration** and the inclusion of **protein-rich foods** can help regulate metabolism and support muscle maintenance, which is essential for overall health.

In some alternative medicine practices, **food as medicine** is not only about healing individual symptoms but also about achieving **overall balance**. For example, in **Traditional Chinese Medicine (TCM)**, foods are often categorized by their warming or cooling effects, and diets are tailored to balance the body's internal energy, or **Qi**. Similarly, in **Ayurvedic medicine**, dietary therapy is based on a person's unique constitution, or **dosha**, with specific foods recommended to promote balance and harmony within the body.

While diet therapy can be an effective tool for improving health and managing various conditions, it is essential to approach it with care. A balanced, nutrient-rich diet is beneficial for most people, but drastic dietary changes should be made under the guidance of a trained healthcare professional, particularly if dealing with chronic health conditions or allergies. In some cases, supplementation may be recommended to ensure that nutritional gaps are filled, especially if certain foods need to be eliminated or reduced.

In conclusion, nutrition and diet therapy in alternative medicine offers a powerful, natural approach to promoting health and healing. By focusing on whole, nutrient-dense foods and making personalized dietary adjustments, individuals can support their bodies' innate ability to heal and maintain optimal health. Whether it's managing chronic disease, supporting mental health, or improving digestion, diet therapy emphasizes the importance of food in maintaining a balanced, healthy life.

Nutritional Approach to Health

A nutritional approach to health focuses on the vital connection between the food we consume and our overall well-being. In alternative medicine, nutrition is viewed not just as a source of sustenance, but as a powerful tool for promoting healing, preventing illness, and maintaining balance in the body. Rather than relying on pharmaceuticals or invasive procedures, this approach uses food as medicine to address a wide range of health concerns—from digestive issues to chronic disease prevention, mental health, and even skin conditions.

One of the fundamental principles of nutritional therapy is **whole-food-based nutrition**, which emphasizes the consumption of minimally processed, nutrient-dense foods. This includes fruits, vegetables, whole grains, lean proteins, and healthy fats. Whole foods are rich in vitamins, minerals, antioxidants, and other essential nutrients that support the body's natural detoxification processes, immune system, and metabolic functions. By focusing on these foods, individuals can nourish their bodies and reduce the risk of developing chronic conditions like heart disease, diabetes, and high blood pressure.

A crucial aspect of a nutritional approach to health is the incorporation of **anti-inflammatory foods**. Chronic inflammation is believed to be at the root of many health issues, from autoimmune diseases to arthritis, cardiovascular disease, and even cancer. Certain foods are known for their natural anti-inflammatory properties, such as **turmeric**, **ginger**, **green leafy vegetables**, **berries**, and **fatty fish** like salmon and mackerel. These foods help reduce inflammation in the body, providing relief for conditions like rheumatoid arthritis and inflammatory bowel disease. **Omega-3 fatty acids**, found in fatty fish and flaxseeds, are especially beneficial in fighting inflammation and supporting brain health.

Another important component of a nutritional approach to health is **gut health**. The digestive system plays a crucial role in overall well-being, as it affects nutrient absorption, immune function, and even mental health. A diet rich in **fiber**, **probiotics**, and **prebiotics** helps maintain a healthy gut microbiome. Probiotic-rich foods like **yogurt**, **kimchi**, and **sauerkraut** contain beneficial bacteria that support digestion and immune function. Prebiotics, found in foods like **garlic**, **onions**, and **bananas**, nourish these beneficial bacteria, promoting a balanced and healthy gut. When the gut microbiome is in balance, the body is better able to digest food, absorb nutrients, and defend against harmful pathogens.

A **low-glycemic diet** is another common nutritional approach used to improve health, particularly for individuals with **insulin resistance**, **prediabetes**, or **type 2 diabetes**. This diet focuses on consuming foods that have a minimal effect on blood sugar levels. Foods like **whole grains**, **legumes**, **non-starchy vegetables**, and **berries** have a low glycemic index, meaning they help maintain stable blood sugar levels and prevent insulin spikes. Reducing the intake of refined carbohydrates and sugary foods is critical for managing blood sugar and reducing the risk of metabolic disorders.

Nutritional therapy also recognizes the significant impact of **micronutrients** on overall health. Vitamins and minerals are essential for many bodily functions, including immune system support, energy production, and the maintenance of healthy skin, bones, and teeth. For example, **vitamin D** is crucial for bone health and immune function, and deficiencies have been linked to various chronic diseases. **Magnesium**, found in foods like **leafy greens**, **nuts**, and **seeds**, supports muscle and nerve function and helps regulate blood pressure. A deficiency in magnesium has been associated with fatigue, muscle cramps, and poor sleep.

Mental health is another area where nutrition plays a pivotal role. **Nutrient-rich diets** can support emotional well-being, reduce symptoms of anxiety and depression, and improve cognitive function. For instance, **omega-3 fatty acids**, found in fish and flaxseeds, are essential for brain health and have been shown to improve mood and cognitive function. **B vitamins**, particularly **B6**, **B12**, and **folate**, are involved in the production of neurotransmitters that regulate mood, and deficiencies in these vitamins have been linked to mental health conditions like depression and anxiety. **Magnesium** and **vitamin D** also play important roles in reducing stress and supporting emotional balance.

In addition to specific nutrients, a **balanced diet** that includes a variety of foods is key to maintaining overall health. Eating a diverse range of whole foods ensures that the body receives all the essential nutrients it needs for proper functioning. Incorporating a variety of colorful fruits and vegetables into the diet provides a broad spectrum of **antioxidants** that protect the body's cells from damage caused by free radicals. Antioxidants, such as **vitamin C**, **vitamin E**, and **beta-carotene**, play a crucial role in protecting the body from oxidative stress and supporting the immune system.

Hydration is another critical aspect of a nutritional approach to health. Drinking enough water throughout the day is essential for digestion, nutrient absorption, and detoxification. **Herbal**

teas like **ginger** and **chamomile** also provide additional health benefits, including reducing inflammation and promoting relaxation. Adequate hydration supports kidney function, helps regulate body temperature, and keeps the skin hydrated and healthy.

Finally, a nutritional approach to health often emphasizes **mindful eating**—the practice of paying attention to the body's hunger and fullness cues, eating slowly, and appreciating the food being consumed. This practice helps individuals cultivate a positive relationship with food, reduce overeating, and improve digestion. Mindful eating encourages individuals to make healthier food choices, listen to their body's needs, and enjoy the experience of eating.

In conclusion, a nutritional approach to health in alternative medicine underscores the importance of food as a tool for promoting healing, preventing disease, and supporting overall wellness. By focusing on whole, nutrient-dense foods, managing inflammation, supporting gut health, and ensuring proper hydration, individuals can optimize their health and prevent chronic conditions. This holistic approach highlights the profound impact that diet and nutrition have on physical, emotional, and mental well-being. Through mindful food choices and personalized dietary plans, nutrition can play a pivotal role in achieving long-term health and vitality.

Diet Therapy Methods

Diet therapy methods in alternative medicine focus on the healing power of food and nutrition to promote health, prevent disease, and manage existing conditions. This approach to health emphasizes using food as a form of medicine, tailoring diets to the specific needs of an individual based on their health conditions, lifestyle, and overall goals. Unlike traditional treatments that may rely heavily on pharmaceuticals, diet therapy focuses on natural, food-based interventions to support the body's innate healing processes.

Detox Diets are among the most commonly used methods in diet therapy. These diets are designed to eliminate toxins from the body and improve overall organ function, particularly the liver, kidneys, and digestive system. Detox diets often emphasize the consumption of **fresh fruits and vegetables**, **water**, and **herbal teas**, while eliminating processed foods, sugar, caffeine, and alcohol. The idea is to give the body a break from potentially harmful substances and provide it with nutrients that help support its natural detoxification processes. Common detoxifying foods include **citrus fruits**, **leafy greens**, and **turmeric**, all of which are known for their antioxidant and anti-inflammatory properties. Although detox diets should be followed with caution and professional guidance, they are often used to improve energy, reduce inflammation, and promote clearer skin.

Anti-inflammatory diets are another popular approach in diet therapy, especially for managing chronic conditions like

arthritis, **heart disease**, and **autoimmune disorders**. Chronic inflammation is believed to contribute to many diseases, and anti-inflammatory diets focus on foods that reduce inflammation in the body. These diets typically include foods like **fatty fish** (rich in **omega-3 fatty acids**), **olive oil**, **turmeric**, **ginger**, **berries**, and **green leafy vegetables**. These foods are known to have natural anti-inflammatory effects that help reduce pain, swelling, and the risk of further health complications. For example, **omega-3 fatty acids** found in fish like salmon and mackerel help lower inflammation markers in the body, providing relief for conditions such as rheumatoid arthritis and inflammatory bowel disease.

Low-glycemic diets are widely used to manage **diabetes** and **insulin resistance**. The goal of a low-glycemic diet is to reduce the impact of foods on blood sugar levels, which can help stabilize insulin and prevent spikes in blood glucose. Foods that have a low glycemic index, such as **whole grains**, **legumes**, **non-starchy vegetables**, and **fruits** with high fiber content, are emphasized in this diet. These foods release sugar into the bloodstream more slowly, preventing sharp increases in blood sugar and helping to maintain stable energy levels throughout the day. By improving blood sugar control, low-glycemic diets are effective in managing **type 2 diabetes** and **pre-diabetes**, while also supporting heart health and weight management.

Elimination diets are another method often used in diet therapy, particularly for individuals with food allergies, intolerances, or sensitivities. These diets work by systematically removing potential trigger foods from the diet and gradually reintroducing them to identify which foods may be causing discomfort or health issues. Common foods eliminated include **gluten**, **dairy**, **soy**, **eggs**, and **nuts**. By removing these foods, the body may experience relief from symptoms like digestive upset, bloating, skin rashes, or fatigue. Once the offending foods are identified, individuals can tailor their diet to avoid these triggers, improving their overall health and quality of life. This method is commonly used to help manage conditions such as **irritable bowel syndrome (IBS)**, **eczema**, and **food allergies**.

Mediterranean diets are often used for **heart health** and **weight management**. This diet, based on the traditional eating habits of people from countries bordering the Mediterranean Sea, emphasizes **healthy fats** like those found in **olive oil**, **nuts**, and **avocados**, as well as **whole grains**, **lean proteins** (especially fish), **vegetables**, and **fruits**. Studies have shown that the Mediterranean diet can reduce the risk of heart disease, improve cholesterol levels, and aid in weight loss. It also has anti-inflammatory effects, supporting overall health and longevity. The Mediterranean diet has become widely recognized for its ability to support **cardiovascular health** and reduce the risk of chronic diseases like **stroke** and **diabetes**.

Plant-based diets focus on the consumption of whole, plant-based foods and are increasingly used to improve overall health and treat chronic conditions. This approach emphasizes **fruits**, **vegetables**, **whole grains**, **legumes**, and **nuts**, while minimizing or eliminating animal products like **meat** and **dairy**. A plant-based diet is rich in fiber, antioxidants, and phytonutrients that promote heart health, reduce cancer risk, and improve digestive health. People following plant-based diets often report improved energy levels, weight management, and reduced inflammation. These diets are particularly beneficial for individuals managing conditions such as **hypertension**, **type 2 diabetes**, and **obesity**, as they focus on foods that are naturally low in unhealthy fats and high in nutrients.

Paleo diets, which are based on the eating habits of our ancient ancestors, focus on **lean meats**, **fish**, **fruits**, **vegetables**, **nuts**, and **seeds**, while excluding processed foods, grains, and dairy.

The idea is to mimic the natural diet of early humans, emphasizing whole, unprocessed foods that provide the body with essential nutrients while avoiding modern foods that are considered harmful, like refined sugars and grains. The Paleo diet has been linked to improved metabolic health, weight loss, and better blood sugar control. However, it's important to ensure proper nutrient balance, as the exclusion of certain food groups can lead to deficiencies if not managed carefully.

Finally, **nutritional therapy** also includes the incorporation of **superfoods**—nutrient-dense foods that are particularly rich in vitamins, minerals, antioxidants, and other health-promoting compounds. Examples of superfoods include **blueberries, kale, chia seeds**, and **spirulina**. These foods can be added to any diet to enhance nutritional intake and support overall health. Superfoods are believed to boost immunity, improve energy levels, support brain function, and protect against chronic diseases like cancer and heart disease.

In conclusion, diet therapy offers a wide range of methods for improving health, preventing disease, and managing chronic conditions through the power of nutrition. By focusing on whole, natural foods and tailoring diets to an individual's specific health needs, diet therapy can support healing, boost energy, reduce inflammation, and promote long-term well-being. Whether through detoxification, managing blood sugar, or supporting heart health, diet therapy is an essential tool in alternative medicine, emphasizing the profound impact food can have on the body's ability to heal and maintain balance.

Understanding Food Therapy

Food therapy is an approach in alternative medicine that uses specific foods and dietary patterns to support health, prevent illness, and address various medical conditions. Rooted in the belief that food is a powerful tool for healing, this practice emphasizes the connection between nutrition and the body's natural ability to restore balance and function. Instead of focusing on conventional drugs or treatments, food therapy works by harnessing the therapeutic properties of natural ingredients to nourish the body and promote optimal wellness.

At the core of food therapy is the idea that different foods have unique properties that can influence the body's internal systems, such as the immune system, digestive system, and metabolism. **Whole, nutrient-dense foods**, including fruits, vegetables, herbs, and whole grains, are used to provide essential vitamins, minerals, antioxidants, and other compounds that support the body's natural healing processes. Unlike processed or refined foods, which may contain artificial additives, sugars, and unhealthy fats, whole foods are seen as the most effective way to fuel the body and prevent disease.

Food therapy often incorporates the use of **herbal remedies** and **spices** that are known for their healing properties. For example, **ginger** is commonly used to treat digestive issues, such as nausea, bloating, and indigestion. It has anti-inflammatory properties that can help reduce pain and improve circulation. **Turmeric**, with its active compound **curcumin**, is another commonly used spice that offers potent anti-inflammatory and antioxidant benefits. It is often used to support joint health, reduce inflammation, and improve digestive health. Both ginger and turmeric, when consumed as part of a regular diet, can help reduce the risk of chronic inflammation and associated diseases, such as arthritis, cardiovascular disease, and even certain cancers.

Nutritional therapy is also central to food therapy, with a focus on providing the body with the right balance of nutrients to support healing and overall health. **Whole grains**, **lean proteins**, and **healthy fats** such as **avocados**, **nuts**, and **olive oil** are commonly incorporated into therapeutic diets to help regulate blood sugar, promote heart health, and support healthy brain function. The **Mediterranean diet**, which is rich in fruits, vegetables, fish, olive oil, and whole grains, is often used as an example of a food therapy approach that supports longevity and helps reduce the risk of chronic diseases, such as heart disease, diabetes, and certain types of cancer.

A key aspect of food therapy is the focus on **gut health**, as it is believed that a healthy digestive system plays a central role in overall well-being. The **gut microbiome**, consisting of trillions of bacteria that reside in the intestines, influences everything from digestion and metabolism to immune function and mental health. Foods that are high in **fiber**, such as fruits, vegetables, and whole grains, support the growth of beneficial gut bacteria, improving digestion and reducing the risk of gastrointestinal issues like **constipation**, **irritable bowel syndrome (IBS)**, and **inflammatory bowel disease (IBD)**. Additionally, **probiotic-rich foods**, such as **yogurt**, **kimchi**, and **sauerkraut**, provide beneficial bacteria that can help restore balance to the gut microbiome and improve overall digestive health.

Food therapy also places a strong emphasis on **detoxification**, using specific foods to help the body eliminate toxins and support the liver's detoxification process. **Citrus fruits** like lemons and oranges are commonly used for their detoxifying effects, as they are rich in vitamin C and antioxidants that support the liver's ability to process and eliminate harmful substances. **Leafy greens** such as spinach, kale, and arugula are also often recommended for detoxification due to their high chlorophyll content, which helps cleanse the blood and remove toxins from the body.

In food therapy, **customized diets** are often created based on an individual's specific health needs. For example, people with **diabetes** may be advised to follow a **low-glycemic diet** that emphasizes foods that do not cause rapid spikes in blood sugar. This diet typically includes whole grains, non-starchy vegetables, and lean proteins while avoiding processed sugars and refined carbohydrates. **Anti-inflammatory diets** are tailored to individuals with chronic conditions such as **rheumatoid arthritis** or **cardiovascular disease**, focusing on foods that reduce inflammation and support heart health, such as fatty fish, nuts, seeds, and olive oil.

Food allergies and **sensitivities** are also addressed through food therapy. For individuals who are intolerant to certain foods, such as **gluten**, **dairy**, or **soy**, food therapy methods include elimination diets and the gradual reintroduction of foods to identify and avoid triggers. By removing these foods from the diet, individuals may experience a reduction in symptoms such as bloating, fatigue, skin rashes, or digestive discomfort. A customized food therapy approach helps ensure that the body receives adequate nutrition while avoiding allergens or irritants.

An integral component of food therapy is **mindful eating**, which encourages individuals to eat with intention, paying attention to their body's hunger cues, food choices, and eating habits. Mindful eating promotes a positive relationship with food, encourages better digestion, and reduces overeating. By practicing mindfulness, individuals can better understand the signals their body is sending and make healthier food choices that align with their health goals.

In conclusion, food therapy offers a holistic and natural approach to healing by using the power of food to restore balance, promote health, and address specific health concerns. By incorporating nutrient-dense, whole foods, anti-inflammatory herbs, and gut-supporting ingredients, food therapy helps optimize the body's ability to heal itself, prevent disease, and improve overall well-being. Whether used to manage chronic conditions, support detoxification, or promote emotional health, food therapy provides a customizable and accessible way to enhance both physical and mental health through diet.

Yoga and Meditation

Yoga and meditation are widely practiced forms of alternative medicine that focus on the mind-body connection, promoting physical health, emotional balance, and spiritual well-being. Both practices have ancient roots, originating in India, and are now integrated into modern wellness routines worldwide. While they are often associated with physical postures and breathing exercises, yoga and meditation go beyond mere physical activity. They offer a holistic approach to health that incorporates mental clarity, stress relief, and emotional resilience.

Yoga is a discipline that involves a combination of physical postures (asanas), breathing techniques (pranayama), and meditation practices designed to improve flexibility, strength, and balance while also calming the mind. There are many different styles of yoga, ranging from more physically demanding forms like **Vinyasa** or **Ashtanga** to gentle, restorative styles such as **Yin** and **Hatha** yoga. Each style offers its own benefits, from increased muscle strength and improved cardiovascular health to greater flexibility and mental relaxation.

The physical benefits of yoga are numerous. Regular practice has been shown to reduce stress, alleviate chronic pain, improve posture, and increase joint mobility. For individuals with conditions like **arthritis**, **back pain**, or **fibromyalgia**, yoga can be an effective way to reduce stiffness, improve range of motion, and promote overall physical health. Research suggests that yoga's emphasis on breath control and mindful movement can help alleviate symptoms of **anxiety**, **depression**, and **insomnia**, by activating the parasympathetic nervous system—the part of the nervous system responsible for relaxation and recovery.

In addition to physical health, yoga also promotes mental clarity and emotional well-being. The practice encourages mindfulness and helps individuals connect with their bodies and breath, fostering a sense of awareness and presence. By focusing on the present moment and disengaging from external stressors, yoga provides a pathway to reducing anxiety, cultivating inner peace, and promoting emotional balance.

Meditation, often practiced in conjunction with yoga, is a technique used to train the mind and develop greater awareness, concentration, and emotional regulation. Meditation is the practice of focusing the mind, usually through controlled breathing or concentration on a particular object or thought, to quiet the constant flow of thoughts and cultivate a state of mental stillness. There are various types of meditation, such as **mindfulness meditation**, **guided meditation**, **mantra meditation**, and **Loving Kindness Meditation (Metta)**, each offering unique benefits depending on an individual's needs.

Mindfulness meditation is one of the most well-known forms and has gained significant attention in recent years for its ability to reduce stress, improve focus, and promote overall well-being. This form of meditation involves focusing on the present moment, observing thoughts, sensations, and emotions without judgment. Mindfulness meditation has been shown to reduce symptoms of **anxiety, depression**, and **post-traumatic stress disorder (PTSD)**, while improving emotional regulation and resilience. It can also improve sleep, reduce chronic pain, and enhance overall mental clarity.

Guided meditation is another approach that involves listening to a trained meditation teacher or audio recording that provides instructions for mental focus and relaxation. This form of meditation is ideal for beginners, as it offers structure and guidance. Many people find that guided meditation helps them relax more deeply and achieve a state of mental peace more easily.

Mantra meditation, on the other hand, involves the repetition of a word, phrase, or sound (called a mantra) to help calm the mind and enhance concentration. The repetitive nature of mantra meditation can help break the cycle of distracting thoughts and foster a deep sense of inner calm and clarity. This technique is often used in **Transcendental Meditation (TM)** and other spiritual practices.

Research has found that regular meditation practice has profound effects on both the mind and the body. Meditation can lower **blood pressure**, reduce **stress hormones** like cortisol, and improve immune system function. It is also associated with increased grey matter in the brain, which plays a role in memory, decision-making, and emotional regulation. Long-term meditation practice can lead to changes in brain structure that promote healthier responses to stress and increased emotional resilience.

When practiced together, yoga and meditation complement each other by offering a comprehensive approach to health. Yoga's physical postures prepare the body for meditation, increasing flexibility and strength while releasing physical tension. Meditation enhances yoga practice by encouraging mental focus and emotional balance. Together, they form a holistic system that addresses physical, emotional, and mental well-being.

In conclusion, yoga and meditation are powerful practices in alternative medicine that foster a deep connection between the mind and body. Whether used for physical health, emotional well-being, or spiritual growth, these practices offer an array of benefits that contribute to a balanced, healthy lifestyle. By promoting relaxation, reducing stress, improving flexibility, and cultivating mental clarity, yoga and meditation serve as accessible and effective tools for enhancing overall health and improving quality of life.

Overview of Yoga

Yoga is a holistic practice that combines physical postures, breathing techniques, and meditation to promote overall health and well-being. Originating in ancient India thousands of years ago, yoga is not just a form of exercise, but a philosophy and lifestyle aimed at achieving balance between the body, mind, and spirit. Over time, yoga has become a widely recognized and practiced method for enhancing physical fitness, reducing stress, and improving mental clarity, with practitioners around the world embracing its benefits.

At its core, yoga emphasizes the connection between breath and movement. The practice includes a series of **asanas** (postures) designed to strengthen, stretch, and align the body. Each asana is typically paired with a specific breathing technique, known as **pranayama**, which helps to oxygenate the body, calm the mind, and increase energy flow. Together, asanas and pranayama create a rhythm of movement that improves circulation, promotes flexibility, and boosts physical strength. As such, yoga is suitable for people of all ages and fitness levels, as modifications can be made to accommodate physical limitations or specific needs.

One of the key benefits of yoga is its ability to improve **flexibility** and **joint health**. Many yoga poses involve deep stretching, which helps to lengthen muscles and increase the range of motion in the joints. Over time, regular practice can reduce stiffness, improve posture, and alleviate tension in areas that often become tight from stress or sedentary lifestyles, such as the shoulders, neck, and lower back. This makes yoga an excellent complement to more strenuous physical activities, as it helps to prevent injury, maintain muscle balance, and promote recovery.

In addition to physical health, yoga is also renowned for its ability to reduce **stress** and improve **mental well-being**. One of the primary ways yoga helps with stress is through its focus on **mindfulness** and the **mind-body connection**. The practice encourages practitioners to be present in the moment, paying close attention to their breath, thoughts, and bodily sensations. This mindfulness component can reduce feelings of anxiety and promote relaxation, as it encourages a break from the constant busyness of daily life. Many studies have shown that regular yoga practice can lower cortisol (the stress hormone) levels, reduce symptoms of depression and anxiety, and improve overall mood.

Yoga's impact on **mental clarity** and **emotional balance** is also significant. Certain styles of yoga, such as **Hatha**, **Vinyasa**, or **Iyengar**, focus on achieving both physical alignment and mental focus. This integration of movement and concentration can foster greater mental resilience, help individuals manage emotional challenges, and enhance cognitive function. Many practitioners report feeling more grounded, focused, and balanced after a yoga session.

The practice of yoga also promotes **deep relaxation** through meditation and breathwork. Many forms of yoga include meditation sessions that help calm the mind and encourage a state of inner peace. Techniques such as **deep breathing**, **visualization**, and **guided meditation** are often used in conjunction with physical postures to facilitate mental relaxation and promote emotional well-being. **Yoga Nidra**, also known as "yogic sleep," is a particularly deep state of relaxation that allows practitioners to rest while remaining mentally aware, making it an effective tool for stress relief and rejuvenation.

Yoga has also gained recognition for its therapeutic applications. Many individuals turn to yoga to help manage or alleviate symptoms of chronic conditions such as **arthritis**, **back pain**, **migraine**, **insomnia**, and **digestive issues**. In these cases, yoga can serve as a complement to conventional treatments, providing relief and improving quality of life. For example, restorative yoga, which uses props to support the body in passive poses, is often used to aid recovery from injury or surgery, and gentle yoga practices can help reduce pain and inflammation associated with conditions like osteoarthritis.

In addition to physical and mental health, yoga has been linked to **enhanced cardiovascular health** and **immune function**. Studies suggest that regular yoga practice can help reduce **blood pressure**, improve **circulation**, and support heart health. Certain poses, such as **downward dog** and **legs up the wall**, encourage venous blood flow and lymphatic drainage, contributing to better circulation and enhanced immune function. Breathing exercises, in particular, can help regulate the autonomic nervous system, supporting better oxygenation of the blood and promoting relaxation.

For those seeking **spiritual growth**, yoga offers a pathway to self-awareness and inner peace. Many forms of yoga, such as **Kundalini** or **Bhakti yoga**, incorporate spiritual elements that help practitioners connect to a deeper sense of purpose and presence. Yoga's focus on balance, mindfulness, and compassion encourages personal growth and self-discovery, often leading to greater alignment with one's values and spiritual beliefs.

In conclusion, yoga is much more than a physical exercise—it is a comprehensive practice that integrates body, mind, and spirit. Whether practiced for its physical benefits, such as flexibility and strength, its mental and emotional effects, like stress reduction and improved mood, or its spiritual components, yoga offers a versatile and holistic approach to health. From beginners to advanced practitioners, yoga can be tailored to suit individual needs and goals, making it an accessible and transformative practice for enhancing overall well-being.

The Science of Meditation

Meditation is an ancient practice that involves focusing the mind and cultivating a state of mental clarity, relaxation, and heightened awareness. While its roots are deeply embedded in spiritual traditions, particularly in Eastern philosophies like Buddhism and Hinduism, modern research has uncovered significant scientific evidence that supports its broad range of health benefits. The science of meditation shows how this practice can profoundly influence both the brain and body, enhancing physical health, mental well-being, and emotional resilience.

One of the most studied aspects of meditation is its ability to affect the **brain**. Brain imaging studies have demonstrated that regular meditation can lead to structural changes in the brain, particularly in areas related to attention, memory, and emotional regulation. For instance, studies have shown that long-term meditators tend to have increased **grey matter** in regions such as the **hippocampus**, which is involved in memory and learning, and the **prefrontal cortex**, which is associated with decision-making, higher cognition, and emotional control. These changes suggest that meditation can enhance cognitive function, improve focus, and increase emotional stability over time.

Additionally, meditation has been shown to increase **brainwave coherence**. Research using EEG (electroencephalogram) has found that meditative states are associated with **alpha** and **theta** brainwaves, which are linked to deep relaxation and a calm, focused mind. Alpha waves are typically present when the mind is relaxed but alert, while theta waves occur during deeper states of relaxation or light sleep. These brainwave patterns indicate that meditation fosters a state of balance between alertness and relaxation, which helps reduce stress and promote mental clarity.

Another key scientific discovery regarding meditation is its impact on **stress** and the body's **stress response system**. Meditation has been shown to lower levels of the stress hormone **cortisol**, which is produced by the adrenal glands during times of stress. Chronic high levels of cortisol are linked to a range of health problems, including **hypertension**, **immune system suppression**, and **anxiety**. By reducing cortisol levels, meditation helps counteract the harmful effects of chronic stress, improving overall health and contributing to a sense of calm and relaxation. Studies have demonstrated that meditation can significantly reduce both **acute stress** and **chronic stress**, making it an effective tool for managing anxiety and stress-related disorders.

Meditation also plays a critical role in **emotional regulation**. Research has shown that mindfulness and meditation techniques help individuals become more aware of their thoughts and emotions, leading to better emotional control. This mindfulness helps practitioners observe their emotions without becoming overwhelmed by them, allowing for more thoughtful responses rather than impulsive reactions. Meditation has been linked to greater **emotional resilience**, improved mood, and a decrease in negative emotional states, such as **depression** and **anxiety**. **Mindfulness meditation**, in particular, is widely used in therapeutic settings to treat a range of mental health issues, including **generalized anxiety disorder (GAD)**, **depression**, and **PTSD**.

The benefits of meditation extend to **physical health** as well. Regular meditation practice has been shown to lower **blood pressure**, improve **heart rate variability**, and enhance overall cardiovascular health. By promoting relaxation and reducing stress, meditation helps reduce the strain on the heart and blood vessels, lowering the risk of **hypertension** and related cardiovascular conditions. Studies suggest that meditation may even improve the health of the **immune system**, enhancing the body's ability to fight off illness and recover from injury. Additionally, meditation has been found to improve sleep quality, helping individuals fall asleep faster and enjoy deeper, more restorative sleep.

Meditation is also linked to improved **pain management**. Research indicates that mindfulness and other meditation techniques can alter the way the brain processes pain, reducing its intensity and emotional impact. Individuals who practice mindfulness meditation have been shown to experience less pain in response to chronic conditions like **fibromyalgia**, **arthritis**, and **migraines**. Meditation can help shift the focus away from pain and reduce the mental and emotional stress that often accompanies it, contributing to an overall improvement in quality of life for those with chronic pain.

The benefits of meditation are not limited to those with specific health conditions. Even individuals without serious medical issues can experience improved overall well-being by incorporating meditation into their daily routine. Meditation helps foster a sense of **inner peace** and **clarity**, which can lead to increased **productivity**, better decision-making, and improved relationships. It also promotes a sense of **mind-body connection**, allowing individuals to feel more grounded and in tune with their physical and emotional states.

While meditation is often seen as a solitary practice, it can also be used in **group settings** or combined with other therapeutic approaches. Practices like **guided meditation** and **loving-kindness meditation** have been shown to improve social connection and promote empathy, helping individuals develop stronger bonds with others. Integrating meditation with physical practices like **yoga** or **tai chi** can also enhance the benefits, as these practices combine mindfulness with physical movement, improving flexibility, balance, and mental clarity.

In conclusion, the science behind meditation reveals its profound impact on the brain, body, and mind. From reducing stress and improving emotional regulation to enhancing cognitive function and supporting physical health, meditation offers a wide range of scientifically supported benefits. Whether practiced for relaxation, mental clarity, pain management, or emotional resilience, meditation provides a powerful and accessible tool for improving health and enhancing quality of life. With continued research, the full range of its therapeutic potential will likely be further explored, offering more people the opportunity to experience its many positive effects.

The Mind-Body Connection

The mind-body connection refers to the profound relationship between a person's mental and emotional states and their physical health. It is based on the understanding that the mind and body are not separate entities but are intricately linked, with the health of one influencing the health of the other. In alternative medicine, the mind-body connection is often viewed as a crucial component of overall well-being. Practices that integrate this connection, such as yoga, meditation, acupuncture, and even herbal medicine, focus on treating both the mind and body together, recognizing the impact that mental and emotional health can have on physical conditions.

One of the most compelling aspects of the mind-body connection is how mental stress can lead to physical health problems. Chronic stress, anxiety, and emotional trauma can manifest in various ways within the body, from muscle tension and headaches to digestive problems and cardiovascular disease. The body's response to stress involves the release of hormones like **cortisol** and **adrenaline**, which trigger the "fight or flight" response. While these hormones are useful in short bursts during acute stress, prolonged exposure to high levels of these stress hormones can weaken the immune system, increase inflammation, and contribute to chronic conditions such as **high blood pressure**, **heart disease**, and **autoimmune disorders**. This physiological response underscores the importance of managing emotional and mental health to prevent long-term physical health issues.

On the flip side, physical health can also influence mental and emotional states. Chronic pain, illness, or even the physical stress of poor posture or lack of movement can lead to feelings of depression, anxiety, and frustration. The brain and nervous system are deeply interconnected with the body's musculoskeletal and circulatory systems, so physical ailments can directly affect mood and emotional well-being. For example, individuals with **chronic pain** conditions, such as **fibromyalgia** or **arthritis**, often experience a decrease in quality of life due to the impact pain has on their mental health. Similarly, those who are physically inactive may experience **low energy**, **irritability**, and **mental fatigue**.

Alternative medicine seeks to harmonize the mind-body connection by using therapies that treat both mental and physical aspects of health. **Mindfulness practices**, such as **meditation** and **deep-breathing exercises**, are widely recognized for their ability to reduce stress and anxiety, promoting relaxation and emotional well-being. These practices focus on the present moment, helping individuals observe their thoughts without judgment and reducing mental clutter that can contribute to stress. Studies have shown that meditation, in particular, can lower **cortisol** levels and help reduce symptoms of **depression**, **anxiety**, and **post-traumatic stress disorder (PTSD)**, making it an effective way to manage mental health.

Yoga is another practice that bridges the mind-body connection by combining physical postures with breath control and mindfulness. Yoga promotes flexibility, strength, and relaxation, while also encouraging awareness of the body's sensations and emotions. Studies have found that yoga can help reduce anxiety, improve mood, and enhance emotional resilience. By focusing on breath and movement, yoga helps activate the parasympathetic nervous system, which counteracts the effects of stress, reduces heart rate, and promotes relaxation. It is often used as a complementary treatment for conditions like **chronic pain, insomnia**, and **stress-related disorders**.

Acupuncture is another alternative therapy that targets the mind-body connection. Rooted in traditional Chinese medicine, acupuncture involves inserting thin needles into specific points on the body to stimulate energy flow and restore balance. Research has shown that acupuncture can help relieve pain, reduce stress, and improve emotional well-being. It is believed to work by releasing endorphins, the body's natural painkillers, and stimulating the release of neurotransmitters that regulate mood and stress. Acupuncture has been used to treat a range of conditions, including **headaches**, **back pain**, and **anxiety**, highlighting its role in promoting balance between the physical and emotional aspects of health.

In addition to physical practices, **herbal remedies** are commonly used in alternative medicine to support the mind-body connection. For instance, herbs like **lavender**, **chamomile**, and **ashwagandha** are known for their calming and stress-reducing properties. Lavender oil is widely used in aromatherapy to help relax the body and mind, reduce anxiety, and improve sleep quality. **Ashwagandha**, an adaptogen, is used to help the body cope with stress, improve mood, and enhance energy levels. By supporting both physical relaxation and mental clarity, these herbs help restore balance and improve overall health.

A strong mind-body connection is also essential for emotional and mental healing. Practices such as **visualization**, **affirmations**, and **guided imagery** are used in alternative therapies to help individuals overcome emotional obstacles and promote positive mental health. Visualization techniques, often incorporated into meditation, encourage individuals to imagine positive outcomes or visualize healing in the body, which has been shown to reduce stress and promote physical healing. Similarly, affirmations—positive statements repeated to challenge negative thought patterns—can help build emotional resilience and improve self-esteem.

In conclusion, the mind-body connection is central to alternative medicine's approach to health, as it emphasizes the importance of both mental and physical well-being in achieving overall health. By recognizing how emotions, stress, and physical health are intertwined, alternative therapies work to restore balance and promote healing in both the mind and body. Whether through yoga, meditation, acupuncture, or herbal medicine, practices that nurture the mind-body connection are increasingly recognized for their effectiveness in improving both physical and emotional health. As research continues to explore the link between the mind and body, the growing acceptance of this integrated approach will likely shape the future of holistic healthcare.

Naturopathic Medicine

Naturopathic medicine is an alternative healthcare system that emphasizes the body's intrinsic ability to heal itself. Rooted in centuries-old traditions, naturopathy combines modern science with natural therapies to treat and prevent a wide range of health issues. It focuses on holistic care, meaning it considers the physical, emotional, and spiritual aspects of a person's well-being, rather than isolating or focusing on a single symptom or disease.

At the core of naturopathic medicine is the **healing power of nature**. Naturopathic practitioners believe that the body, when given the proper nutrients, environment, and care, is capable of maintaining health and overcoming disease. This philosophy leads to treatments that support and enhance the body's natural processes rather than suppressing symptoms with pharmaceuticals. Practitioners aim to identify and address the root causes of illness rather than just alleviating the symptoms.

Naturopathy uses a wide range of natural therapies to restore balance and promote healing, including **herbal medicine, nutrition, hydrotherapy, homeopathy, acupuncture**, and **physical medicine. Herbal medicine** is one of the cornerstones of naturopathy, with practitioners using plants and plant extracts to treat illnesses. Common herbs like **echinacea, ginger, turmeric**, and **chamomile** have long been used for their healing properties, ranging from boosting immunity to reducing inflammation.

Nutrition therapy is also central to naturopathy. Naturopathic doctors emphasize the importance of a balanced, nutrient-rich diet in supporting the body's natural ability to heal. They often recommend individualized nutritional plans, which may include the use of **vitamin and mineral supplements**, **detox diets**, and **elimination diets**. For example, patients with conditions like **diabetes** or **heart disease** may be advised to adopt diets rich in whole grains, healthy fats, and lean proteins, while limiting refined sugars and processed foods.

Another key treatment in naturopathic medicine is **hydrotherapy**, which uses water in various forms—such as hot or cold compresses, saunas, or hydrotherapy baths—to stimulate circulation, relieve pain, and promote detoxification. Hydrotherapy is often used for conditions like **muscle soreness**, **arthritis**, or **digestive issues**, as it helps to improve circulation and reduce inflammation.

Homeopathy, though a more controversial approach within the broader field of alternative medicine, is sometimes incorporated into naturopathic practices. Homeopathy involves the use of highly diluted substances to trigger the body's self-healing mechanisms. Homeopaths believe that tiny doses of a substance that causes symptoms in a healthy person can, in turn, cure those same symptoms in a sick person. While research on the efficacy of homeopathy remains mixed, some patients report positive results, particularly for chronic conditions such as **allergies** or **mild digestive issues**.

Acupuncture, which is rooted in Traditional Chinese Medicine (TCM), is also commonly integrated into naturopathic care. Acupuncture involves inserting thin needles into specific points on the body to stimulate energy flow, improve circulation, and alleviate pain. Naturopathic doctors use acupuncture to treat conditions like **chronic pain**, **migraines**, and **stress**. By balancing the body's energy flow, acupuncture helps restore harmony to the body's systems, supporting the body's innate healing abilities.

Physical medicine therapies are often used in conjunction with other naturopathic treatments. These may include **massage therapy**, **spinal manipulation**, and **exercise prescriptions** to promote mobility, reduce pain, and support musculoskeletal health. Many naturopathic doctors are also trained in **osteopathic techniques**, which focus on treating the body as a whole and using physical manipulation to enhance overall health.

One of the key principles in naturopathic medicine is **patient-centered care**. Naturopaths take the time to listen to their patients, understand their lifestyles, and develop personalized treatment plans. This individualized approach not only addresses the physical symptoms but also incorporates factors like stress, emotional health, and lifestyle habits. Naturopathic practitioners often encourage patients to adopt preventive measures, such as regular exercise, stress reduction practices (like meditation or yoga), and sufficient sleep, to maintain long-term health.

A core belief of naturopathic medicine is that prevention is just as important as treatment. Naturopathic doctors aim to help patients achieve **optimal wellness** by teaching them how to make healthier lifestyle choices and take responsibility for their health. This focus on prevention can help reduce the risk of chronic conditions, such as **heart disease**, **diabetes**, and **autoimmune disorders**. By focusing on overall health and well-being rather than just the treatment of disease, naturopathy encourages patients to maintain a balance between physical health, mental wellness, and emotional resilience.

While naturopathic medicine is widely used and valued by many patients for its holistic approach, it is important to note that it is not without controversy. Critics argue that some of the treatments, such as homeopathy, lack scientific evidence to support their effectiveness. As with any form of alternative medicine, it is important for patients to work with qualified, licensed practitioners and consider combining naturopathy with conventional medicine for comprehensive care, particularly in the case of serious or life-threatening conditions.

In conclusion, naturopathic medicine is a comprehensive, patient-centered approach to health that focuses on natural healing, prevention, and the body's ability to maintain balance. By incorporating a variety of therapies, such as herbal medicine, nutrition, acupuncture, and hydrotherapy, naturopathy aims to treat the root causes of illness and support long-term wellness. While it may not replace conventional medicine in all cases, it offers a valuable complement to traditional healthcare and provides individuals with the tools and knowledge to maintain optimal health in a holistic, sustainable way.

Principles of Naturopathy

Naturopathy is an alternative medicine system that emphasizes the body's innate ability to heal itself. It operates on a set of core principles that guide the treatment of illness and the promotion of health. These principles integrate natural therapies, such as herbal medicine, nutrition, hydrotherapy, and lifestyle changes, to support both the body and mind in achieving optimal health. Rather than focusing on the mere alleviation of symptoms, naturopathy seeks to identify and address the root causes of illness and imbalances in the body.

One of the fundamental principles of naturopathy is the **healing power of nature**. Naturopaths believe that the body has a powerful innate ability to heal itself, given the right conditions. By supporting the body with proper nutrition, rest, and natural therapies, the healing process is optimized. This principle emphasizes **natural, non-invasive treatments**, such as herbal remedies, proper diet, and physical treatments, to enhance the body's own healing processes. Naturopaths often encourage a lifestyle that fosters balance, vitality, and long-term health, rather than relying on drugs or invasive procedures.

The principle of **treating the whole person** is another key aspect of naturopathy. Naturopaths focus not only on the physical symptoms of a disease but also consider a person's emotional, mental, and spiritual well-being. This holistic approach involves addressing the interconnectedness of the body's systems, rather than isolating and treating symptoms in isolation. For example, a naturopathic treatment plan might include dietary adjustments, herbal supplements, and mindfulness practices to address stress, poor sleep, or other emotional factors that may contribute to physical ailments. The aim is to balance the body, mind, and spirit, fostering overall well-being.

Identifying and treating the root cause of illness is a core tenet of naturopathy. Rather than simply masking symptoms, naturopaths strive to uncover the underlying imbalances or factors that contribute to a person's health condition. This might involve addressing lifestyle factors, environmental toxins, or emotional stressors that could be affecting physical health. For instance, a patient suffering from chronic digestive issues may not just be given medication for relief but might also undergo an evaluation of their diet, stress levels, and gut health to identify what is causing the imbalance. By treating the root cause, naturopathy aims to prevent the recurrence of illness and promote long-term health.

Another central principle is **the prevention of disease**. Naturopathic medicine places a strong emphasis on **preventative care**, teaching patients how to maintain good health through balanced nutrition, regular exercise, and stress management. Naturopaths encourage lifestyle choices that enhance the body's natural resistance to disease and help individuals maintain a state of health, rather than waiting until an illness develops. This principle supports the idea that health is not simply the absence of disease but a dynamic state of well-being, achieved through proactive, daily habits.

First, do no harm is a guiding principle in naturopathy, meaning that naturopathic practitioners strive to use treatments that are gentle, non-toxic, and minimally invasive. The therapies employed in naturopathy, such as herbal medicine, acupuncture, or dietary changes, are considered safer and more natural alternatives to pharmaceutical interventions or surgical procedures. In cases where conventional treatments are necessary, naturopaths may refer patients to other healthcare professionals to ensure the most appropriate care.

Doctor as teacher is another important principle in naturopathy. Naturopathic practitioners view themselves not just as healers but as educators who empower patients to take an active role in their health and wellness. This principle emphasizes the importance of educating patients about their own bodies, the causes of disease, and how to make healthier lifestyle choices. By fostering a greater understanding of health, naturopaths aim to help patients adopt habits that support long-term wellness, such as improving nutrition, reducing stress, and incorporating physical activity into their daily lives.

Vitalism is another foundational principle of naturopathy, which states that the body is an interconnected system of vital energy or force. This vital force, often referred to as "life energy" or **Qi** in Traditional Chinese Medicine, is believed to drive the body's physiological functions and maintain balance. When the vital force is compromised or imbalanced, disease can manifest. Naturopathic treatments are designed to restore and strengthen the body's vital force, allowing for the natural healing process to take place.

Finally, **treatment with the least force** emphasizes the use of the most gentle, effective treatments possible. Naturopathic medicine values the use of natural therapies that work with the body rather than forcing or overriding its natural processes. Whether through **dietary changes**, **herbal remedies**, **massage therapy**, or **exercise**, the goal is to gently guide the body toward health without causing harm or disruption to its natural balance.

In conclusion, the principles of naturopathy reflect a holistic approach to health that integrates natural healing, preventative care, and a deep respect for the body's intrinsic ability to heal itself. By treating the whole person, addressing the root cause of illness, and empowering patients to take control of their health, naturopathy offers a comprehensive, natural alternative to conventional medicine. These guiding principles continue to inspire and shape the practice of naturopathic medicine, offering patients a path to long-term wellness and vitality.

Therapies and Treatments

Alternative medicine encompasses a wide range of therapies and treatments that focus on natural healing, balance, and the body's innate ability to restore itself. These treatments often prioritize individualized care, aiming to treat the whole person—body, mind, and spirit—rather than just addressing symptoms. Below are some of the most widely recognized therapies within alternative medicine and their unique approaches to health and healing.

Herbal medicine is one of the oldest forms of alternative therapy, with plants and plant-based substances used for medicinal purposes for thousands of years. Herbal remedies can support a wide variety of health conditions, from boosting immunity to reducing inflammation and alleviating digestive issues. For example, **echinacea** is commonly used to enhance immune function and ward off colds, while **ginger** is often used for its anti-inflammatory properties and ability to ease nausea. Herbal medicine can be used in many forms, including teas, tinctures, capsules, and topical applications, and is often integrated with other forms of alternative treatment.

Acupuncture is a central treatment in Traditional Chinese Medicine (TCM), where thin needles are inserted into specific points on the body, called **acupoints**, to stimulate energy flow, or **Qi**. The goal is to restore balance and promote healing by unblocking any energy stagnation in the body. Acupuncture is often used to treat conditions like **chronic pain**, **headaches**, **stress**, and **insomnia**. It is believed that stimulating these acupoints helps to release endorphins, improve circulation, and balance the nervous system, aiding in the body's self-healing processes.

Chiropractic care focuses on the alignment of the spine and musculoskeletal system, with the belief that proper alignment helps the body function optimally. Spinal adjustments, also known as **spinal manipulation**, are used to correct misalignments (known as **subluxations**) that may lead to pain, inflammation, or limited mobility. Chiropractors use hands-on techniques to improve spinal function and alleviate symptoms related to **back pain**, **neck pain**, and **headaches**. Chiropractic therapy often involves a combination of spinal adjustments, physical therapy, and lifestyle recommendations to improve health.

Massage therapy is a widely used method for promoting relaxation, reducing stress, and alleviating muscle tension. There are various types of massage, including **Swedish**, **deep tissue**, **shiatsu**, and **sports massage**, each with a specific focus and therapeutic goal. Massage therapy works by manipulating the muscles and soft tissues of the body to improve circulation, relieve muscle stiffness, and reduce stress. Regular massage is also known to enhance lymphatic drainage, support immune function, and promote emotional well-being by lowering cortisol levels and increasing endorphin production.

Homeopathy is a system of alternative medicine that uses highly diluted substances to stimulate the body's healing response. The principle behind homeopathy is **"like cures like"**—that is, a substance that causes symptoms in a healthy person can, in small doses, cure similar symptoms in a sick person. Homeopaths select remedies based on a person's individual symptoms and overall constitution, considering both physical and emotional factors. While the scientific evidence supporting homeopathy remains controversial, many individuals find it useful for addressing chronic conditions, **allergies**, **digestive issues**, and **sleep disturbances**.

Aromatherapy involves the use of essential oils from plants to promote physical and emotional well-being. These oils can be inhaled, applied topically, or used in massage to alleviate stress, enhance mood, and treat various ailments. For example, **lavender oil** is known for its calming effects, often used to reduce anxiety and promote restful sleep. **Peppermint oil** can be used to relieve headaches, muscle tension, and digestive discomfort. Aromatherapy works by stimulating the olfactory system, which is closely linked to the brain's limbic system, responsible for regulating emotions and memory.

Naturopathy is a holistic system of medicine that focuses on supporting the body's self-healing mechanisms through natural treatments. Naturopaths use a combination of therapies, including **nutrition**, **herbal medicine**, **hydrotherapy**, **homeopathy**, and **physical medicine**, to treat both acute and chronic conditions. Naturopathy emphasizes the importance of lifestyle changes, such as a healthy diet, regular exercise, and stress management, to maintain balance and prevent illness. Naturopathic practitioners treat the underlying causes of disease rather than merely masking symptoms, aiming to address physical, emotional, and environmental factors that contribute to poor health.

Mind-body therapies are practices that promote physical and mental well-being by focusing on the mind's influence over the body. Techniques such as **meditation**, **yoga**, **guided imagery**, and **biofeedback** are commonly used to reduce stress, improve mental clarity, and promote relaxation. Meditation helps by quieting the mind and focusing attention, which can lower blood pressure, improve heart rate variability, and reduce symptoms of anxiety and depression. Yoga combines physical postures with breath control and mindfulness to promote flexibility, strength, and inner peace, while also reducing stress and improving emotional balance.

Energy healing therapies, such as **Reiki**, **Qi Gong**, and **Therapeutic Touch**, are based on the belief that the body has an energy field that can be balanced and restored to improve health. Energy healing involves the practitioner channeling healing energy into the patient's body, aiming to release blockages and restore balance to the energy flow. While the scientific evidence for energy healing is still evolving, many people report significant improvements in relaxation, pain relief, and emotional well-being after receiving treatments.

Detoxification is a practice in alternative medicine that involves cleansing the body of accumulated toxins, often through dietary changes, fasting, or the use of herbal supplements. Detox programs aim to support the liver, kidneys, and digestive system in their natural detoxification processes. Common detox strategies include **juice cleanses**, **herbal detox teas**, and **colon hydrotherapy**. Detoxification is believed to enhance energy levels, improve skin health, and support the immune system by removing harmful substances from the body.

In conclusion, the therapies and treatments in alternative medicine offer a wide range of approaches to improving health and wellness. Whether through **herbal remedies**, **spinal adjustments**, **energy healing**, or **mind-body techniques**, these therapies are designed to promote balance, enhance the body's self-healing capacity, and support long-term health. Many of these treatments are used in conjunction with conventional medical care, providing a holistic and complementary approach to health.

The Role of a Naturopathic Doctor

A naturopathic doctor (ND) is a licensed healthcare professional who focuses on using natural, holistic treatments to support the body's ability to heal and maintain health. Naturopathy combines modern medical science with centuries-old natural healing practices, aiming to treat the whole person—body, mind, and spirit. The role of a naturopathic doctor is diverse, as they are trained to diagnose, prevent, and treat a wide range of health conditions using natural remedies, lifestyle changes, and integrative medicine.

One of the core tenets of naturopathic medicine is the belief in the **body's inherent ability to heal itself**. Naturopathic doctors focus on strengthening the body's natural healing mechanisms, rather than simply treating symptoms. They take a **patient-centered approach**, considering each individual's unique health history, lifestyle, genetics, and emotional well-being. By identifying the root causes of illness, naturopathic doctors create personalized treatment plans aimed at restoring balance and health.

Diagnosis and treatment are integral parts of a naturopathic doctor's role. Like conventional medical doctors, NDs perform thorough physical exams, take medical histories, and order diagnostic tests when necessary. However, they are also trained to assess other factors such as nutrition, lifestyle, environmental influences, and emotional health, which could contribute to a patient's condition. This comprehensive approach allows naturopathic doctors to address the root cause of illness rather than just managing symptoms.

Naturopathic treatments often include **natural therapies** like **herbal medicine, nutrition, hydrotherapy, acupuncture**, and **homeopathy**. NDs may recommend **dietary adjustments** to improve health, such as incorporating more whole foods, eliminating processed foods, or identifying food sensitivities. Herbal remedies are frequently prescribed to boost the immune system, alleviate inflammation, or address specific health concerns. **Hydrotherapy** (the use of water for healing) might be suggested to improve circulation or detoxify the body, while **acupuncture** may be used to help manage pain or balance energy within the body. **Homeopathic remedies**, though controversial in some medical circles, are also used by NDs for their belief in stimulating the body's vital force to restore health.

Beyond these specific therapies, a naturopathic doctor plays an important role in **preventative care**. Prevention is a cornerstone of naturopathic medicine, with NDs focusing on helping patients maintain optimal health rather than merely treating illness after it occurs. This preventative approach includes lifestyle counseling, stress management techniques, sleep hygiene recommendations, and advice on physical activity, all of which contribute to long-term well-being. By addressing lifestyle factors that contribute to disease, NDs aim to reduce the risk of developing chronic conditions like heart disease, diabetes, and autoimmune disorders.

Naturopathic doctors also educate patients about the importance of **self-care**. They empower individuals to take control of their health by teaching them how to make informed decisions about nutrition, exercise, and mental health. This emphasis on patient education helps foster a partnership between doctor and patient, where the patient becomes an active participant in their own healing process. NDs may also recommend stress-reducing techniques, like yoga, meditation, or mindfulness, to help patients cope with emotional or psychological stress, which can have significant effects on physical health.

In addition to the physical aspects of healing, naturopathic doctors recognize the significance of **emotional and mental health**. They take a holistic approach by acknowledging how stress, emotional trauma, and mental health challenges can manifest as physical symptoms. As part of their treatment plan, NDs may incorporate **mind-body therapies**, including meditation, guided imagery, or relaxation exercises, to help patients reduce stress and improve mental clarity. This integration of the mind-body connection is a key element in the naturopathic philosophy of treating the whole person.

In some cases, a naturopathic doctor may work alongside conventional medical practitioners, providing complementary care. For example, an ND might collaborate with an oncologist to help a cancer patient manage side effects from chemotherapy using nutrition and herbal remedies. This integrative approach allows patients to benefit from both conventional treatments and the natural therapies provided by naturopathy. In these situations, open communication between healthcare providers is essential to ensure safe and effective care.

It's important to note that naturopathic medicine is not a replacement for conventional medicine in all situations. Naturopathic doctors are trained to recognize when a patient requires conventional treatments, such as surgery or emergency care, and will refer patients to specialists when necessary. NDs are particularly effective in managing **chronic conditions**, **preventive care**, and **lifestyle-related diseases**, where natural therapies can support and enhance conventional treatments.

In conclusion, naturopathic doctors play a pivotal role in alternative medicine by offering a holistic, patient-centered approach to health and healing. By combining natural remedies, lifestyle counseling, and preventative care, NDs help patients improve their physical, mental, and emotional well-being. Whether treating specific health conditions or fostering long-term wellness, naturopathic medicine provides a comprehensive, integrative approach that focuses on the body's inherent ability to heal itself.

Ayurvedic Medicine

Ayurvedic medicine is an ancient system of healing that originated in India over 3,000 years ago. Rooted in the philosophy that health is a state of balance between the body, mind, and spirit, Ayurveda offers a holistic approach to wellness. The term **Ayurveda** comes from the Sanskrit words "Ayur" meaning life and "Veda" meaning knowledge, thus translating to "the knowledge of life." This comprehensive system uses a combination of dietary changes, herbal remedies, body therapies, meditation, and lifestyle adjustments to promote harmony within the body and prevent disease.

One of the fundamental principles of Ayurveda is the belief in the **three doshas**, or life forces, which are thought to govern the body's functions and health. These doshas are **Vata**, **Pitta**, and **Kapha**, and each person is believed to have a unique balance of these three energies, which influences their physical and mental characteristics. **Vata** is associated with movement and governs bodily functions such as circulation, breathing, and nerve impulses. **Pitta** is linked to transformation and controls digestion, metabolism, and energy production. **Kapha** is associated with structure and stability, managing growth, lubrication, and immune function. By understanding one's dosha, an Ayurvedic practitioner can recommend personalized treatments that restore balance and optimize health.

Ayurvedic treatments focus on **restoring balance** to the doshas and enhancing the body's natural healing abilities. **Dietary changes** are an important aspect of Ayurveda, with foods categorized based on their qualities, such as hot or cold, heavy or light, and moist or dry. For example, individuals with a predominance of **Pitta** (often associated with fiery energy) may be advised to eat cooling foods, such as dairy, cucumbers, and leafy greens, to calm the digestive system and avoid overheating. Conversely, individuals with **Vata** imbalances (associated with dryness and cold) may be encouraged to consume grounding and warming foods, like cooked grains and root vegetables.

In addition to dietary recommendations, **herbal medicine** plays a central role in Ayurvedic therapy. Herbs are used to restore balance, detoxify the body, and promote healing. Popular Ayurvedic herbs include **turmeric**, which has anti-inflammatory and antioxidant properties; **ashwagandha**, known for its stress-reducing and adaptogenic qualities; and **triphala**, a blend of three fruits used to improve digestion and detoxify the body. These herbs are often prepared as powders, teas, or capsules, depending on the individual's needs.

Ayurvedic medicine also emphasizes the importance of **detoxification**. The process of **Panchakarma** is one of the most widely recognized Ayurvedic detox treatments. Panchakarma is a series of therapeutic procedures designed to cleanse the body of accumulated toxins (known as **ama**) and rejuvenate the body's tissues. The treatment involves various steps, including **oil massages**, **herbal steam baths**, and **medicated enemas**, all tailored to an individual's dosha and health condition. This detoxification process is believed to improve digestion, increase energy, and promote overall well-being.

Beyond physical treatments, Ayurveda also emphasizes the role of **mental health** in achieving overall balance. Practices such as **meditation**, **yoga**, and **breathing exercises** (pranayama) are often recommended to calm the mind, reduce stress, and restore harmony. Ayurvedic medicine teaches that emotional well-being is closely tied to physical health, and therefore mental practices are integrated into the healing process. Meditation, in particular, helps cultivate mindfulness and self-awareness, allowing individuals to better understand their thoughts and emotions, and how these impact their physical health.

Lifestyle practices are another cornerstone of Ayurveda. The daily routine, known as the **Dinacharya**, is recommended to maintain balance and health. This routine includes activities such as waking up early, practicing gentle yoga, following a consistent eating schedule, and engaging in self-care rituals like **oil massage** (Abhyanga). These practices are tailored to an individual's dosha, lifestyle, and health conditions, promoting a balanced life and long-term wellness.

One of Ayurveda's most important aspects is its focus on **preventive care**. Rather than simply treating diseases, Ayurveda encourages individuals to adopt healthy habits that prevent illness and maintain optimal well-being. This proactive approach emphasizes the importance of understanding one's unique body constitution and making lifestyle and dietary choices that promote balance. Regular Ayurvedic treatments, such as oil massages, detoxification, and meditation, can help individuals maintain health and prevent disease.

While Ayurveda has been practiced for thousands of years and has provided relief for countless individuals, it is important to approach it with an open mind and proper guidance. Ayurvedic medicine is best practiced under the supervision of a qualified practitioner who can assess an individual's dosha and health needs, and tailor treatments accordingly. Like any form of alternative medicine, it's important to ensure that Ayurvedic practices are used alongside conventional medical care, particularly for serious or acute health conditions.

In conclusion, Ayurvedic medicine offers a holistic, individualized approach to health that emphasizes balance between the body, mind, and spirit. By using natural treatments like herbal remedies, dietary adjustments, detoxification, and lifestyle practices, Ayurveda aims to restore harmony and promote long-term wellness. Its focus on prevention, personalization, and overall balance makes it a valuable complement to conventional medicine, particularly for those seeking natural, preventive, and comprehensive care.

Concept of Ayurveda

Ayurveda is a comprehensive system of medicine that originated in ancient India over 3,000 years ago. It is based on the understanding that health is the result of a balance between the body, mind, and spirit, and that disease arises when this balance is disrupted. The word "Ayurveda" itself comes from two Sanskrit words: "Ayur," meaning life, and "Veda," meaning knowledge or science, thus translating to the "science of life." Ayurveda focuses on maintaining health and preventing disease rather than merely treating symptoms, emphasizing a holistic approach that integrates the physical, mental, and spiritual aspects of well-being.

One of the central concepts in Ayurveda is the idea of the **three doshas**—**Vata**, **Pitta**, and **Kapha**—which are the fundamental energies or principles that govern the body's functions. These doshas are made up of the five elements (earth, water, fire, air, and ether) and are present in different proportions in each individual. Vata is associated with air and ether and governs movement, including circulation and breathing. Pitta, associated with fire and water, controls digestion, metabolism, and energy production. Kapha, made from earth and water, is responsible for structure, lubrication, and immune function.

Each person has a unique constitution, or **Prakriti**, which is the specific combination of these doshas at the time of their birth. Understanding one's dosha is essential for maintaining balance and health, as an imbalance in any of the doshas can lead to illness. For example, if **Vata** becomes too dominant, it may lead to conditions like anxiety, dryness, or digestive issues, while an excess of **Pitta** can result in inflammation, anger, or digestive disturbances. **Kapha** imbalances might manifest as sluggishness, weight gain, or respiratory issues. Ayurveda aims to restore the natural balance of the doshas through a combination of diet, lifestyle changes, herbal medicine, and other therapies.

Another key concept in Ayurveda is **Agni**, or digestive fire. According to Ayurvedic principles, digestion is the foundation of good health. A strong Agni is believed to promote proper digestion, assimilation of nutrients, and elimination of waste, while a weak or imbalanced Agni can lead to poor digestion, toxins in the body (referred to as **Ama**), and the development of disease. Ayurveda places significant emphasis on maintaining a balanced diet and proper digestion as essential for overall health.

Ojas, the vital energy that sustains life, is also a fundamental concept in Ayurveda. It is believed that a person's physical, mental, and emotional well-being is supported by Ojas. A deficiency in Ojas can lead to fatigue, weakened immunity, and susceptibility to disease. Maintaining balance through proper diet, lifestyle practices, and emotional well-being is thought to nourish and protect Ojas, leading to vitality and resilience.

Detoxification is another core element of Ayurvedic practice. The process of **Panchakarma**, a detoxifying treatment, aims to remove toxins from the body and restore balance. It involves a series of therapeutic procedures such as **oil massages**, **steam therapy**, **herbal enemas**, and other purification techniques. The goal of Panchakarma is to cleanse the body of **Ama** (toxins) and restore the balance of the doshas, which can promote rejuvenation, enhance energy levels, and improve overall health.

Diet is a central pillar in Ayurvedic medicine. Ayurvedic dietary recommendations are based on an individual's dosha, current health condition, season, and climate. Foods are categorized according to their properties, such as hot, cold, dry, or moist, and are matched to balance an individual's constitution and current needs. For example, individuals with a **Pitta** imbalance, which is associated with excess heat and inflammation, may be advised to eat cooling foods like cucumbers, dairy, and leafy greens, while individuals with a **Kapha** imbalance might benefit from lighter, spicier foods to stimulate digestion and reduce excess fluid retention.

In addition to diet and herbal medicine, **Ayurvedic lifestyle practices** play a significant role in health and longevity. These practices include **Dinacharya** (daily routine), which emphasizes consistent sleep, exercise, and work habits; **Ritucharya** (seasonal routine), which adjusts lifestyle and diet according to the changing seasons; and **Sattvic** practices, which encourage mental clarity, peacefulness, and ethical living. These principles align daily life with the rhythms of nature, supporting harmony and balance within the body.

Herbal remedies are widely used in Ayurveda to treat a wide range of conditions, from digestive issues and inflammation to mental health concerns. Common herbs used in Ayurvedic medicine include **Ashwagandha**, an adaptogen that helps combat stress and promote vitality; **Turmeric**, known for its anti-inflammatory properties; and **Tulsi** (Holy Basil), which is revered for its immune-boosting and stress-reducing effects. These herbs are used in various forms, such as powders, teas, capsules, and oils, depending on the individual's needs.

Ayurveda also recognizes the importance of **mental and emotional health**. The practice of **meditation**, **yoga**, and **breathing exercises** (pranayama) is often incorporated into Ayurvedic treatment plans to balance the mind and emotions.

Meditation helps reduce stress, improve focus, and promote emotional clarity, while yoga postures help enhance physical flexibility and strength, promote proper circulation, and calm the mind.

In conclusion, Ayurveda offers a comprehensive, holistic approach to health that seeks to restore balance to the body, mind, and spirit. By understanding the unique constitution of each individual, Ayurveda tailors treatments to help achieve optimal wellness and prevent disease. Through diet, herbal remedies, lifestyle changes, and mind-body practices, Ayurveda promotes a balanced life and supports the body's natural ability to heal itself. As a system of medicine deeply rooted in nature, Ayurveda continues to be an important and effective approach to health and healing in the modern world.

Ayurvedic Practices

Ayurvedic practices are a cornerstone of Ayurvedic medicine, aiming to restore balance and harmony between the body, mind, and spirit. Rooted in ancient wisdom, these practices focus on achieving holistic wellness by emphasizing natural, preventive, and personalized healing methods. Ayurveda approaches health as an individualized experience, where lifestyle, diet, and environment all play significant roles in maintaining or restoring balance. The goal is to optimize the body's natural healing abilities, prevent disease, and promote long-term vitality.

One of the key Ayurvedic practices is the **daily routine**, known as **Dinacharya**, which encourages consistency and balance in everyday life. By following a daily routine that aligns with natural rhythms, individuals can maintain physical, mental, and emotional well-being. Practices within Dinacharya include waking up early, preferably before sunrise, to begin the day with meditation or mindfulness. Morning rituals also often include drinking warm water to stimulate digestion and performing **oil pulling** with sesame or coconut oil to detoxify the mouth and improve oral health. Regularity in sleep, eating, and physical activity is encouraged, as well as maintaining a calm and peaceful mindset throughout the day.

Dietary practices are at the heart of Ayurveda, as food is considered both nourishment and medicine. According to Ayurvedic principles, the foods you eat should be tailored to your unique constitution (dosha) and current imbalances. Foods are classified by their qualities—such as hot, cold, dry, or oily—and are used to balance the doshas. For example, individuals with **Pitta** (which is associated with heat and intensity) may be advised to consume cooling foods such as cucumbers, dairy, and leafy greens, while those with **Kapha** (which is associated with cold and dampness) might benefit from lighter, spicier foods like peppers and ginger to stimulate digestion and balance excess moisture in the body.

An important Ayurvedic practice is the concept of **detoxification**, often referred to as **Panchakarma**. This therapeutic process aims to cleanse the body of toxins (known as **Ama**) and restore balance by eliminating accumulated waste and impurities. Panchakarma involves a series of treatments, including **oil massages** (Abhyanga), **herbal steam baths**, **nasal irrigation** (Nasya), and **medicated enemas** (Vasti), to detoxify the body and rejuvenate the mind. The specific treatments used in Panchakarma are tailored to an individual's dosha, current health condition, and seasonal needs. These therapies help balance the doshas, improve digestion, and strengthen the immune system, promoting optimal health and well-being.

Herbal remedies are another essential aspect of Ayurvedic practices. Ayurvedic medicine relies on the healing properties of herbs to address imbalances in the body. Herbs such as **turmeric**, **ashwagandha**, **holy basil (Tulsi)**, and **ginger** are commonly used in Ayurvedic treatments for their anti-inflammatory, adaptogenic, and immune-boosting properties. Herbal formulations, often in the form of teas, powders, tinctures, or capsules, are designed to address specific health concerns, including digestive issues, stress, immune function, and skin health. These remedies are considered powerful tools to restore balance within the body and support its natural healing processes.

In Ayurveda, **massage therapies** play a crucial role in maintaining physical and mental health. The practice of **Abhyanga**, or Ayurvedic oil massage, is designed to detoxify the body, promote circulation, and balance the doshas. Warm herbal oils, often infused with healing herbs, are used to massage the body, promoting relaxation and rejuvenation. This practice is thought to improve blood circulation, remove toxins, reduce stress, and enhance mental clarity. Additionally, **Shirodhara**, a form of Ayurvedic treatment involving the pouring of warm oil over the forehead, is used to calm the nervous system, relieve stress, and improve mental clarity.

Breathing exercises (pranayama) and **meditation** are also integral parts of Ayurvedic practices that contribute to overall well-being. Pranayama is a system of controlled breathing techniques used to regulate the flow of **prana** (life energy) in the body, calm the mind, and promote mental clarity. Specific techniques like **Nadi Shodhana** (alternate nostril breathing) are used to balance the body's energy and reduce stress. Meditation, often practiced alongside pranayama, helps calm the mind, improve concentration, and promote emotional well-being. Both pranayama and meditation are designed to enhance spiritual awareness and emotional resilience, supporting the body's ability to maintain balance and health.

Ayurveda also incorporates **seasonal routines**, or **Ritucharya**, which align lifestyle and diet with the changing seasons. Seasonal shifts can bring about imbalances in the body, and Ayurvedic practices adjust to these changes by recommending specific foods, activities, and self-care practices to keep the doshas in harmony with the environment. For example, during the cold winter months, Ayurvedic practices recommend warm, grounding foods and activities to nourish and energize the body, while during the hot summer months, cooling and hydrating foods like cucumbers and melons are recommended to calm excessive heat in the body.

Lastly, Ayurvedic medicine emphasizes the importance of maintaining a **balanced mind** through practices that nurture mental health and emotional stability. Ayurveda recognizes that mental and emotional health significantly impacts physical health. Therefore, practices like **mindfulness**, **yoga**, and **journaling** are encouraged to help manage stress, promote emotional healing, and cultivate a positive outlook. Ayurveda places great importance on **Sattva**—the state of mental clarity and calm—and suggests lifestyle adjustments that can help foster peace of mind, reduce negative emotions, and support overall mental health.

In conclusion, Ayurvedic practices offer a deeply holistic approach to health, focusing on personalized care, natural healing, and balance in all aspects of life. Whether through dietary recommendations, herbal remedies, detoxification, massage, or mental health practices, Ayurveda seeks to restore harmony and vitality by treating the whole person—body, mind, and spirit. These practices provide powerful tools for maintaining long-term health and preventing illness, making Ayurveda a valuable and comprehensive system of alternative medicine.

The Three Doshas

In Ayurvedic medicine, the concept of the **three doshas**—**Vata**, **Pitta**, and **Kapha**—is central to understanding health and disease. These doshas are the fundamental energies believed to govern the body and mind, and each individual has a unique combination of them, which influences their physical, emotional, and mental characteristics. The balance of these doshas determines a person's health and well-being, and an imbalance in any of them is thought to lead to disease or discomfort. The key to maintaining health in Ayurveda lies in understanding your dosha and managing its balance.

Vata is the dosha associated with movement and is made up of the elements **air** and **ether** (space). It governs processes like circulation, breathing, nerve impulses, and the movement of thoughts in the mind. People with a **Vata** constitution are typically energetic, creative, and quick-thinking, but when out of balance, they can become anxious, restless, or suffer from digestive issues like constipation or bloating. **Vata** individuals are often thin, with dry skin, and they may be more susceptible to conditions related to dryness, such as arthritis or insomnia. To balance **Vata**, Ayurveda recommends warm, moist foods, regular routines, and grounding practices like yoga or meditation. Since **Vata** tends to increase with cold weather, the colder months may exacerbate **Vata** imbalances, which is why **Vata** types should avoid cold, raw foods and opt for warming, nourishing dishes.

Pitta, the dosha of transformation, is composed of **fire** and **water** elements. It governs digestion, metabolism, body temperature, and energy production. People with a **Pitta** constitution are typically intense, focused, and assertive. They tend to have strong digestion and a robust immune system, but when out of balance, **Pitta** types can become irritable, overheated, and prone to inflammation, acid reflux, or skin conditions like acne or rashes. **Pitta** individuals are often medium-built with warm, oily skin, and they thrive in moderate temperatures. To balance **Pitta**, Ayurveda recommends cooling, calming foods, like dairy, cucumbers, and leafy greens. Avoiding spicy, fried, and overly salty foods, which can aggravate **Pitta**, is also important. As **Pitta** is often heightened in hot climates, the summer months are a time when **Pitta** imbalances may occur, and cooling practices are beneficial during this time.

Kapha is the dosha associated with structure and stability, made up of the elements **earth** and **water**. It governs the physical structure of the body, such as the bones, muscles, and tissues, as well as fluid balance, immunity, and lubrication. People with a **Kapha** constitution tend to have a sturdy, strong build, with smooth skin and often a calm, steady demeanor. **Kapha** types are generally calm, loving, and grounded but may become sluggish, possessive, or gain weight easily when **Kapha** is out of balance. They may suffer from congestion, respiratory issues like asthma, or conditions related to excess moisture, such as sinus infections. To balance **Kapha**, Ayurveda recommends stimulating, light, and dry foods, such as leafy greens, beans, and spices like ginger, turmeric, and black pepper. Reducing intake of dairy and fatty foods, as well as increasing physical activity, is important to keep **Kapha** in check, especially during the cold and damp winter months when **Kapha** energy tends to increase.

Each person has a unique combination of these doshas, known as their **Prakriti**, which is determined at birth. This inherent constitution influences how they respond to food, climate, exercise, and stress. Ayurvedic practitioners assess an individual's dosha type by observing physical characteristics, habits, mental tendencies, and imbalances. Through this personalized approach, Ayurveda offers tailored recommendations for diet, lifestyle, and treatments that can help restore balance to the body and mind.

The balance of the doshas is also influenced by the **season**, **age**, and **lifestyle**. For example, **Vata** increases during the fall and early winter, **Pitta** peaks in summer, and **Kapha** is more pronounced during spring. Understanding these seasonal shifts can help individuals modify their diet and lifestyle to maintain balance and prevent imbalances during certain times of the year.

In summary, the three doshas—**Vata**, **Pitta**, and **Kapha**—are fundamental to understanding health in Ayurveda. Each dosha represents a different aspect of life energy, and their balance or imbalance influences every aspect of a person's well-being, from physical health to emotional states. By identifying your dosha and understanding how it affects you, Ayurveda offers personalized approaches to diet, lifestyle, and therapy, promoting harmony within the body and mind. Balancing the doshas is essential for achieving optimal health, vitality, and longevity.

Energy Medicine

Energy medicine is an alternative healing modality that focuses on balancing and restoring the body's energy fields to promote health and well-being. Based on the concept that the body is not only a physical structure but also an energetic system, energy medicine seeks to address imbalances or blockages in the body's energy flow, which can contribute to illness or discomfort. Practitioners believe that by working with these energy fields, health can be restored, symptoms alleviated, and the body's natural healing abilities activated.

One of the most well-known forms of energy medicine is **Reiki**, a Japanese practice that involves the practitioner channeling universal energy into the patient's body through their hands. The belief is that this energy flow can promote relaxation, reduce stress, and accelerate the body's healing process. Reiki practitioners use a light touch or no touch at all, placing their hands on or near specific areas of the body, with the intent to guide energy where it is needed. The practice has been reported to help with pain relief, improve emotional well-being, and support recovery from various health conditions.

Another widely practiced form of energy medicine is **acupuncture**, which is rooted in Traditional Chinese Medicine. Acupuncture involves the insertion of very thin needles into specific points along the body's meridian pathways to stimulate energy flow, or **Qi**. This practice is based on the belief that disruptions or blockages in the flow of Qi can cause illness. By inserting needles into strategic points, acupuncture aims to restore balance, alleviate pain, and enhance the body's natural ability to heal. Acupuncture has been used to treat a wide range of conditions, including chronic pain, stress, digestive issues, and even insomnia.

Healing Touch is another form of energy medicine where practitioners use their hands to clear, energize, and balance the human energy field. It involves techniques that may include gentle touch, near-body work, and visualization. The aim is to restore the proper flow of energy, reduce pain, and promote physical and emotional healing. Healing Touch is often used in hospitals and healthcare settings to help manage pain, reduce stress, and support recovery in patients with chronic conditions or undergoing surgery.

EFT (Emotional Freedom Techniques), also known as tapping, is an energy medicine technique that combines elements of **acupuncture** with cognitive therapy. The practice involves tapping on specific points on the body, primarily along the meridian lines, while focusing on a specific issue or emotional blockage. It is believed that tapping on these points can help release negative emotions, reduce stress, and shift the body's energy patterns, leading to emotional and physical healing. EFT is commonly used for conditions such as anxiety, PTSD, and chronic pain.

One important concept in energy medicine is the **human biofield**, which refers to the energy field surrounding and permeating the body. This biofield is thought to be responsible for maintaining physical and emotional health, and disruptions in its balance are believed to contribute to disease. Many forms of energy healing, such as Reiki and Healing Touch, work to manipulate or clear the biofield to restore health. The biofield is sometimes visualized as an electromagnetic field that can be measured through devices like the **Bioptron light therapy** or

Kirlian photography, which capture images of the body's energy.

Quantum Healing is another aspect of energy medicine that draws on principles of quantum physics, where practitioners believe that consciousness and energy interact to influence the physical body. Quantum healing emphasizes the power of intention, belief, and mind-body connection in the healing process. It suggests that by shifting energy patterns at a quantum level, significant changes can occur in the body's health, and healing can take place on both a physical and spiritual level. This form of energy medicine often integrates visualization, meditation, and other techniques to help realign the body's energy system.

Energy medicine also intersects with **crystal healing**, which involves using gemstones and crystals that are believed to have specific energetic properties. These stones are thought to influence the body's energy field and restore balance. Different types of crystals are said to promote various healing properties, such as **amethyst** for emotional healing, **rose quartz** for love and compassion, and **clear quartz** for clarity and healing. Crystals are often used during meditation, placed on the body, or worn as jewelry to support energy flow and promote wellness.

While energy medicine is based on principles that may seem abstract or difficult to measure scientifically, numerous studies and anecdotal evidence suggest that energy healing can have positive effects on physical, emotional, and mental health. Many people report feeling relaxed, rejuvenated, and emotionally lighter after receiving energy treatments. Some practitioners also believe that energy medicine can accelerate healing from illness and injury by removing energetic blockages and fostering a state of balance and vitality.

In conclusion, energy medicine offers a unique and holistic approach to health, focusing on the subtle energy systems that govern the body. Whether through Reiki, acupuncture, Healing Touch, or other techniques, energy medicine seeks to restore balance to the body's energy field, promote self-healing, and enhance well-being. While it may be considered a complementary treatment to conventional medicine, many individuals find it helpful in reducing stress, alleviating pain, and improving emotional health. The practice of energy medicine highlights the connection between mind, body, and spirit, offering a deeper understanding of how energy influences health and healing.

The Field of Energy Medicine

Energy medicine is a field within alternative medicine that focuses on the concept of energy as a central component of human health and healing. This field operates on the premise that the human body is not just a physical structure but also an intricate system of energy fields that influence both physical and emotional health. Energy medicine practitioners work with these energy fields—often referred to as biofields—to balance, restore, and optimize the body's natural flow of energy, which is believed to promote healing and overall well-being.

At the core of energy medicine is the idea that disruptions or imbalances in the body's energy flow can lead to illness, disease, or emotional distress. Just as the body is made up of physical systems like the circulatory and nervous systems, it is also believed to possess an energetic system that maintains harmony and health. This energy is often referred to as **Qi** (in Traditional Chinese Medicine), **Prana** (in Ayurveda), or simply as the **biofield** in scientific terms. Energy medicine seeks to detect and correct these imbalances through a variety of therapeutic techniques.

One of the most well-known practices in energy medicine is **acupuncture**, a fundamental component of Traditional Chinese Medicine (TCM). Acupuncture involves the insertion of fine needles into specific points on the body, called **acupoints**, along pathways known as **meridians**. These meridians are believed to conduct energy throughout the body. Acupuncture aims to restore balance and unblock stagnant energy (Qi) to alleviate pain, improve circulation, and support the body's self-healing processes. The practice is commonly used to treat conditions like **chronic pain, stress, digestive issues**, and **sleep disorders**.

Another prominent form of energy medicine is **Reiki**, a Japanese healing practice in which a practitioner uses their hands to channel universal energy into the patient's body. The goal is to balance the patient's energy field and promote relaxation, reduce stress, and accelerate the body's natural healing processes. Reiki is commonly used for relaxation, emotional healing, and pain management, and can be performed with or without physical touch. Reiki practitioners believe that energy flows through the hands, targeting areas of the body that are energetically blocked or depleted.

Healing Touch is an energy therapy that involves the practitioner using their hands to interact with the energy field of the body. This gentle, non-invasive technique helps clear, balance, and energize the human biofield. Healing Touch practitioners use a variety of hand positions on or above the body to remove energetic blockages, promote relaxation, and enhance the body's ability to heal. It is often used to help alleviate **stress**, **pain**, **anxiety**, and **depression**. Healing Touch is sometimes integrated with conventional medical care to support recovery from surgeries, injuries, and chronic illness.

Emotional Freedom Techniques (EFT), also known as tapping, is another energy medicine practice that combines elements of **acupuncture** with cognitive therapy. It involves tapping on specific acupressure points on the body while focusing on particular emotional issues or physical symptoms. EFT is based on the idea that tapping on these points while addressing negative emotions can release energy blockages, reduce the intensity of emotional responses, and alleviate physical discomfort. EFT has gained popularity as a self-help tool for reducing **stress, anxiety, trauma,** and **pain**.

Quantum Healing is a form of energy medicine that combines concepts from quantum physics and energy medicine. It proposes that consciousness and energy influence the body's physical state and that healing can occur by altering energy patterns at a quantum level. Quantum healing emphasizes the power of the mind and intention in the healing process. By shifting energy patterns through meditation, visualization, or intention-based therapies, practitioners believe that individuals can facilitate deep healing and transformation in both the body and mind.

The concept of the **biofield** is another important element in energy medicine. The biofield refers to the energy field that surrounds and permeates the human body. While it is not directly visible, scientists and practitioners believe that this field influences the physical body's health and can be measured with various biofeedback technologies. The biofield interacts with other energy systems, including the electromagnetic field, which the body generates. By promoting the balance of the biofield, energy medicine practitioners aim to support the body's ability to maintain health, resist disease, and heal from illness or injury.

Energy medicine also includes practices such as **crystal healing**, which involves using gemstones or crystals to influence the body's energy field. Different crystals are believed to have distinct energetic properties that can address specific health concerns. For example, **amethyst** is used for emotional healing, while **clear quartz** is often used to enhance energy flow and promote clarity. Crystals are typically used in conjunction with other energy therapies like meditation or

Reiki, and are either placed on the body or held during healing sessions.

One of the primary goals of energy medicine is to restore the body's natural **energetic balance**. Energy imbalances or blockages can manifest as physical ailments, emotional distress, or a general sense of disconnection from one's well-being. By addressing these imbalances, energy medicine seeks to alleviate symptoms, promote healing, and foster a sense of harmony within the body. It is often used as a complementary treatment alongside conventional medical care to support recovery, reduce side effects of treatment, and promote overall wellness.

Energy medicine practices are increasingly being used in **integrative medicine** settings, where they are combined with traditional medical treatments to support patient recovery, reduce stress, and improve emotional health. Many hospitals and healthcare centers now offer energy healing therapies, such as Reiki or Healing Touch, alongside conventional treatments for cancer, surgery recovery, or pain management.

In conclusion, the field of energy medicine is based on the idea that energy plays a crucial role in the body's health and healing processes. Through therapies such as acupuncture, Reiki, Healing Touch, EFT, and crystal healing, energy medicine works to restore balance and optimize the body's energy flow. While it is often used in conjunction with conventional medicine, energy medicine offers a unique and holistic approach to health that addresses not just the physical body but the energetic systems that influence overall well-being.

Techniques and Treatments

Alternative medicine includes a wide range of techniques and treatments designed to promote healing, improve well-being, and prevent illness by addressing the root causes of health problems. These approaches often prioritize natural, non-invasive methods that work with the body's innate healing abilities. Here are some of the most commonly used techniques and treatments in alternative medicine, each offering unique benefits for physical, emotional, and mental health.

One of the most widely recognized techniques in alternative medicine is **acupuncture**. Rooted in Traditional Chinese Medicine (TCM), acupuncture involves inserting thin, sterile needles into specific points along the body's meridians, or energy pathways, to stimulate the flow of **Qi** (energy). Acupuncture is used to address a variety of conditions, including **chronic pain**, **stress**, **headaches**, **digestive issues**, and **insomnia**. The goal is to restore balance to the body's energy, relieve blockages, and promote overall healing. Research has shown that acupuncture can help improve circulation, release endorphins, and enhance the body's natural healing processes.

Chiropractic care is another popular alternative treatment focused on the alignment of the spine and musculoskeletal system. Chiropractors use **spinal manipulation** (or adjustments) to correct misalignments, also known as

subluxations, that are thought to interfere with the nervous system. By realigning the spine, chiropractic adjustments can help relieve pain, reduce inflammation, and improve function, particularly for those suffering from back pain, neck pain, and headaches. In addition to spinal adjustments, chiropractors often recommend exercises, stretching, and lifestyle modifications to support long-term health.

Massage therapy involves the manipulation of soft tissues, such as muscles, tendons, and ligaments, to promote relaxation, improve circulation, and alleviate pain. There are several different types of massage, including **Swedish massage**, **deep tissue massage**, **Shiatsu**, and **sports massage**, each with its own techniques and benefits. Regular massage therapy can help reduce stress, relieve muscle tension, improve joint flexibility, and enhance overall well-being. It is often used as a complementary therapy for conditions like **chronic pain**, **muscle injuries**, **arthritis**, and **stress-related disorders**.

Herbal medicine is another cornerstone of alternative medicine. It involves using plants, herbs, and plant-based extracts for therapeutic purposes. Many common herbs, such as **ginger**, **turmeric**, **chamomile**, and **peppermint**, have well-established health benefits, such as reducing inflammation, aiding digestion, and promoting relaxation. Herbal medicine can be used in various forms, including teas, tinctures, capsules, and topical applications. It is often used to address conditions like **digestive issues**, **respiratory problems**, **skin conditions**, and **immune system support**. However, it's important to consult a healthcare professional to ensure the safe use of herbs, especially when combining them with conventional medications.

Homeopathy is a holistic treatment approach based on the principle of "like cures like," which asserts that substances that cause symptoms in a healthy person can, in small doses, treat similar symptoms in a sick person. Homeopathic remedies are highly diluted versions of natural substances such as plants, minerals, or animals. The remedies are prescribed based on the individual's specific symptoms and constitution, with the goal of stimulating the body's self-healing response. Homeopathy is commonly used for conditions like **allergies, migraine headaches, digestive issues**, and **skin conditions**. While some studies suggest its efficacy, homeopathy remains a controversial practice due to the lack of strong scientific evidence supporting its effectiveness.

Aromatherapy involves the use of essential oils extracted from plants to enhance physical and emotional well-being. These oils are often inhaled, massaged into the skin, or used in diffusers to create therapeutic effects. Different essential oils are believed to have specific properties, such as **lavender** for relaxation, **peppermint** for energy, and **eucalyptus** for respiratory health. Aromatherapy is used to address conditions such as **stress, anxiety, headaches**, and **sleep disorders**. Many people find it helpful in creating a calming environment and managing everyday stress.

Reiki is a Japanese technique used to reduce stress and promote healing by channeling energy through the hands of a practitioner into the patient's body. It is based on the belief that a universal life force energy flows through all living things and that disruptions in this energy can lead to illness. Reiki practitioners use their hands to direct energy to areas of the body where energy is blocked or out of balance. This non-invasive therapy is often used to enhance relaxation, support emotional healing, and alleviate pain or stress. It is commonly applied to help individuals with **chronic pain, anxiety, depression**, and **fatigue**.

Energy healing therapies, such as **Healing Touch** or **Therapeutic Touch**, work on the premise that the body's energy field plays a vital role in health. Practitioners of energy healing work by gently placing their hands near or on the body, clearing blockages in the biofield, and restoring the flow of energy. This can result in relaxation, reduced pain, and an improved sense of well-being. Energy healing is often used to treat stress-related conditions, emotional trauma, chronic pain, and fatigue.

Dietary therapies are also widely used in alternative medicine to treat and prevent disease. These therapies emphasize the consumption of whole, nutrient-dense foods and the elimination of processed, refined, and unhealthy foods. For instance, an **anti-inflammatory diet** may be recommended to reduce chronic inflammation associated with conditions like **arthritis** or **cardiovascular disease**, while a **detox diet** may be used to support the liver and kidneys in eliminating toxins from the body. **Nutritional supplements**, such as vitamins, minerals, and probiotics, may also be recommended to address deficiencies or imbalances.

Finally, **mind-body techniques** like **meditation**, **yoga**, and **breathing exercises** are widely practiced in alternative medicine to reduce stress, enhance mental clarity, and promote emotional well-being. Meditation involves quieting the mind and focusing on the present moment, while yoga combines physical postures with breathing exercises to improve flexibility, strength, and mental focus. These practices have been shown to reduce stress, lower blood pressure, improve mood, and promote overall health. They are commonly used in conjunction with other therapies to enhance healing and improve quality of life.

In conclusion, the diverse array of techniques and treatments in alternative medicine offers individuals a holistic approach to health and healing. Whether through physical therapies like acupuncture and massage, natural remedies like herbal medicine, or mind-body practices like yoga and meditation, alternative medicine focuses on restoring balance and supporting the body's natural ability to heal itself. Many people find these therapies valuable for managing chronic conditions, reducing stress, and maintaining long-term well-being.

Understanding Qi and Meridians

In Traditional Chinese Medicine (TCM), **Qi** (pronounced "chee") is considered the vital life force or energy that flows through all living things. It is believed to be the fundamental force that sustains life and is responsible for all physical and mental processes. Qi is not a tangible substance but an energetic flow that influences the body's function, health, and balance. In TCM, the flow of Qi is paramount, and any disruptions or imbalances in its movement are thought to lead to disease and illness.

Qi flows through the body along specific pathways known as **meridians**. These meridians are like energetic highways that connect various organs and systems of the body, allowing the free flow of Qi. There are **12 main meridians** in the body, each corresponding to a specific organ system, such as the **liver**, **heart**, **lungs**, and **kidneys**. Each of these meridians is also paired with another meridian to create a balanced system of energy throughout the body. For example, the **lung meridian** is paired with the **large intestine meridian**, and the **heart meridian** is paired with the **small intestine meridian**.

The concept of meridians and Qi flow is the foundation of practices such as **acupuncture**, **acupressure**, and **herbal medicine** in Traditional Chinese Medicine. Acupuncture, for instance, involves inserting thin needles at specific points along the meridians to restore balance and facilitate the smooth flow of Qi. If Qi is blocked, stagnant, or deficient in any of the meridians, it can result in symptoms or health problems, such as pain, digestive issues, or emotional imbalances. By stimulating certain acupoints along the meridians, practitioners can remove blockages and encourage Qi to flow freely, thereby promoting healing and restoring balance.

In addition to the 12 primary meridians, there are **extraordinary meridians**, which are less well-known but play a vital role in maintaining the overall balance of energy within the body. These meridians are thought to store and regulate Qi, and they act as a reservoir to help redistribute energy when needed. They are closely linked to the body's most important functions and are often involved in the treatment of chronic or complex conditions.

The proper flow of Qi is said to support the body's **physical health** and **emotional well-being**. TCM believes that when Qi is flowing smoothly and harmoniously, a person feels balanced, healthy, and energized. Conversely, when the flow of Qi is obstructed, weak, or excessive, it can lead to health problems, both physical and emotional. **Stagnant Qi** might cause conditions such as pain, tightness, or swelling, while **excessive Qi** can lead to symptoms like restlessness, inflammation, or high blood pressure. **Deficient Qi** is associated with fatigue, weakness, or a weakened immune system. The goal in TCM is to maintain a balanced flow of Qi throughout the body to prevent and treat illnesses.

Meridian therapy involves the use of techniques such as **acupuncture, acupressure, cupping,** and **moxibustion** to influence the flow of Qi and address imbalances in the body. **Acupuncture** involves inserting needles at specific acupoints along the meridians to stimulate Qi flow, while **acupressure** uses finger pressure on the same points. **Cupping** therapy involves creating suction on the skin to improve blood flow and release stagnant Qi, and **moxibustion** uses the heat from burning herbs, typically **mugwort**, to warm specific acupoints and promote the movement of Qi.

Meridian theory also emphasizes the importance of **balance** between the body's Yin and Yang energies, which are the complementary forces that represent opposite but interconnected aspects of life. Yin is associated with qualities such as coolness, rest, and nourishment, while Yang represents warmth, activity, and vitality. In this framework, Qi moves between these two forces to maintain equilibrium in the body, mind, and spirit. Disruptions in the balance of Yin and Yang can affect the flow of Qi and result in illness.

In addition to acupuncture and physical therapies, **herbal remedies** are also used to regulate Qi and the meridians. Herbs in TCM are believed to have specific energetic properties—cooling, warming, drying, or moistening—that can help restore balance to the meridians and the flow of Qi. For example, **ginseng** is often used to invigorate the Qi and boost energy, while **licorice root** is known to harmonize the body and strengthen the flow of Qi.

In summary, Qi and meridians are foundational concepts in Traditional Chinese Medicine that provide a framework for understanding how the body functions energetically. Qi, the vital life force, flows through the meridians, influencing all aspects of health, from physical vitality to emotional balance. By using therapies such as acupuncture, acupressure, and herbal medicine, practitioners aim to restore the free flow of Qi and maintain the body's harmony and balance. Whether addressing pain, digestive issues, or emotional distress, understanding and working with Qi and meridians is a key part of promoting health and healing in alternative medicine.

Integrative Medicine

Integrative medicine is an approach to healthcare that combines conventional medical treatments with alternative therapies to address the full spectrum of a patient's physical, emotional, mental, and spiritual health. Unlike conventional medicine, which often focuses solely on treating disease or symptoms, integrative medicine emphasizes a holistic approach to wellness. The goal is to support the body's natural ability to heal itself while incorporating the best practices from both conventional and alternative medicine to enhance patient outcomes.

In integrative medicine, practitioners work collaboratively with patients, combining evidence-based conventional treatments—such as surgery, prescription medications, or physical therapy—with complementary practices such as **acupuncture**, **herbal medicine**, **mind-body techniques**, and **nutrition therapy**. This multi-faceted approach allows for personalized treatment plans that not only target the symptoms of illness but also address underlying causes and promote overall health and well-being.

One of the core principles of integrative medicine is **patient-centered care**. This approach places the patient at the center of their healthcare, recognizing that every individual is unique and requires a personalized treatment plan. Practitioners of integrative medicine take the time to understand the patient's health history, lifestyle, values, and preferences, using this information to tailor their treatment approach. This model encourages open communication between patients and healthcare providers, creating a strong partnership for achieving long-term wellness.

Mind-body techniques are a key aspect of integrative medicine, as they focus on the interconnectedness of the mind and body. Practices like **meditation, yoga, guided imagery**, and **deep-breathing exercises** are used to help manage stress, reduce pain, and promote emotional healing. For example, **mindfulness-based stress reduction (MBSR)** has been shown to improve chronic pain management, reduce anxiety, and enhance overall quality of life. These techniques work by helping patients tap into their inner resources to better cope with physical and emotional challenges.

Acupuncture, an ancient therapy from Traditional Chinese Medicine, is often used in integrative medicine to help manage pain, enhance recovery, and restore balance in the body's energy systems. By inserting thin needles into specific points along the body's meridians, acupuncture aims to stimulate the body's natural healing mechanisms. Studies have shown that acupuncture can be effective in treating a variety of conditions, including **musculoskeletal pain, headaches**, and **stress**.

Another important aspect of integrative medicine is the use of **nutrition therapy** to support healing and overall health. A balanced, nutrient-dense diet is often seen as a foundational aspect of health, and in integrative medicine, nutrition is tailored to support the body's unique needs. For example, patients with chronic illnesses like **diabetes** or **heart disease** may be advised to adopt specific dietary plans, such as a **low-glycemic** or **Mediterranean diet**, to improve their health and manage their condition. Integrative practitioners also emphasize the role of **supplements** like **vitamins, minerals**, and **herbal remedies** to address deficiencies and promote healing.

Herbal medicine is frequently incorporated into integrative care to complement conventional treatments. Herbs like **ginger**, **turmeric**, and **echinacea** are often used for their anti-inflammatory, immune-boosting, and pain-relieving properties. However, integrative medicine practitioners use these remedies in conjunction with conventional medications and therapies, ensuring that the herbs support the body's healing process without interfering with other treatments. This synergy between herbal remedies and conventional medicine can enhance patient recovery and improve health outcomes.

Chiropractic care is another component of integrative medicine, particularly for conditions related to the musculoskeletal system, such as **back pain**, **neck pain**, or **headaches**. Chiropractors use hands-on spinal adjustments to align the spine and restore proper nervous system function. This approach can complement conventional treatments by improving mobility, reducing pain, and enhancing overall physical function.

While integrative medicine combines conventional and alternative therapies, it also emphasizes **prevention** and **wellness**. Practitioners often work with patients to develop lifestyle plans that promote long-term health, including regular physical activity, stress management techniques, and preventive screenings. This preventative approach aims to address risk factors before they develop into serious health conditions, helping patients maintain their health and avoid illness in the future.

For integrative medicine to be effective, collaboration between different healthcare providers is essential. **Medical doctors, naturopathic doctors, chiropractors, acupuncturists, nutritionists**, and other practitioners often work together to develop an individualized treatment plan that combines the best aspects of both conventional and alternative medicine. This team-based approach ensures that patients receive the most comprehensive care possible, with each practitioner bringing their unique expertise to the table.

In conclusion, integrative medicine represents a comprehensive approach to healthcare that combines the best of conventional and alternative therapies. By focusing on the whole person—addressing physical, mental, and emotional health—integrative medicine offers a more personalized, holistic path to wellness. Whether through the use of acupuncture, nutrition therapy, mind-body practices, or herbal remedies, integrative medicine aims to not only treat symptoms but also prevent illness, support healing, and improve overall well-being. This approach has gained increasing recognition for its ability to provide effective, patient-centered care that enhances the quality of life and supports long-term health.

Integrative vs Alternative Medicine

In the world of healthcare, both integrative and alternative medicine offer unique approaches to health and healing, often contrasting with conventional medical practices. While they share some commonalities, such as a focus on holistic treatment and non-invasive therapies, they differ significantly in their philosophy, scope, and application. Understanding the distinctions between these two forms of treatment can help individuals make informed decisions about their healthcare options.

Alternative medicine refers to therapies and practices that are used in place of conventional medicine. These approaches are often rooted in traditional healing systems or new-age methods that prioritize natural, non-pharmaceutical solutions to health issues. In many cases, alternative medicine practitioners treat conditions without the use of drugs or surgery, instead relying on herbal remedies, acupuncture, homeopathy, and energy therapies, among others.

One of the defining characteristics of alternative medicine is its **independence from mainstream medical practices**. Alternative treatments often operate outside the established medical system and may not be subject to the same rigorous testing and regulation as conventional drugs and therapies. For example, herbal remedies, though widely used, are not always backed by the same level of scientific evidence as pharmaceuticals. While some alternative therapies like **acupuncture** or **herbal medicine** have gained recognition for their therapeutic benefits, others, like **homeopathy**, remain controversial due to limited empirical support.

On the other hand, **integrative medicine** blends conventional medical practices with alternative therapies in a **coordinated and collaborative** manner. Rather than replacing traditional medicine, integrative medicine works alongside it, offering a more comprehensive approach to healthcare. Integrative practitioners draw from a variety of disciplines, including **conventional medicine, naturopathy, chiropractic care, acupuncture, mind-body therapies**, and **herbal medicine**, depending on the patient's needs and preferences. The goal of integrative medicine is to address not only physical symptoms but also emotional, mental, and spiritual well-being, promoting overall health and balance.

A key difference between integrative and alternative medicine lies in their **relationship with conventional medicine**. While alternative medicine often positions itself as an alternative to mainstream healthcare, integrative medicine seeks to **integrate** these practices. Integrative medicine recognizes the value of conventional medical treatments, such as surgery, prescription medications, and diagnostic testing, and incorporates complementary therapies to enhance their effectiveness. For instance, a person undergoing cancer treatment might receive chemotherapy or radiation from a conventional oncologist while also working with an acupuncturist or nutritionist to manage side effects, improve quality of life, and support overall well-being.

In practice, **integrative medicine** tends to focus more on collaboration between healthcare providers. Medical doctors, naturopathic doctors, acupuncturists, massage therapists, and other practitioners work together to create a comprehensive treatment plan that balances both conventional and alternative approaches. This collaborative model allows for a more personalized approach, as treatments are tailored to each individual's unique health needs and preferences. It also provides patients with access to a wider range of therapeutic options, all while ensuring that conventional treatments are not overlooked or abandoned.

In contrast, **alternative medicine** may be practiced independently, with individuals opting for therapies outside of the conventional medical framework. While some alternative medicine practitioners are open to collaboration with conventional doctors, others may reject mainstream medicine altogether, preferring to treat conditions entirely with natural remedies. This independence can sometimes lead to a lack of integration, where patients may receive treatment that is disconnected from conventional care or may not be fully informed about potential interactions between alternative and conventional therapies.

The scope of treatment in **integrative medicine** also tends to be broader, incorporating a **preventive approach** that focuses not just on treating existing health problems, but also on promoting wellness and preventing disease. Integrative practitioners often guide patients in lifestyle modifications that support long-term health, such as improved diet, exercise, stress management, and sleep hygiene. Alternative medicine, while often focusing on symptom relief or addressing specific conditions, may not always emphasize the same preventive aspects.

In terms of evidence-based practice, integrative medicine places a strong emphasis on the use of **scientifically-supported therapies**. It combines the best of both worlds, incorporating alternative practices that have been shown to have therapeutic benefits with the reliability and efficacy of conventional medicine. Alternative medicine, while it may incorporate evidence-based practices such as acupuncture or herbal remedies, often includes therapies that have less scientific validation or are still considered experimental in the wider medical community.

In conclusion, the key difference between integrative and alternative medicine lies in their **approach to conventional healthcare**. Integrative medicine combines the strengths of both conventional and alternative practices, providing a holistic, personalized approach to treatment and prevention. It emphasizes collaboration between various healthcare providers, with the goal of optimizing health and well-being. **Alternative medicine**, while offering valuable treatments, tends to operate outside the conventional medical system and often focuses on natural, non-pharmaceutical interventions as standalone treatments. Both approaches have their place in the broader landscape of healthcare, with integrative medicine offering a more collaborative and inclusive path to healing.

The Scope of Integrative Care

Integrative care is a holistic approach to healthcare that blends conventional medicine with complementary and alternative therapies to address the full range of a person's health needs. It acknowledges the importance of treating not only the physical symptoms of illness but also the emotional, mental, and spiritual aspects of well-being. The scope of integrative care is broad, as it involves a comprehensive treatment plan that combines the best of both worlds—conventional medicine and alternative treatments—to optimize health and healing.

One of the core principles of integrative care is **personalized treatment**. Every individual has a unique set of health concerns, lifestyle factors, and personal preferences. Integrative care recognizes this individuality and tailors treatment plans accordingly. Whether someone is managing a chronic illness, recovering from surgery, or simply aiming to improve overall wellness, an integrative care approach takes the time to consider the full spectrum of health needs. This often involves working with a team of healthcare professionals who specialize in both conventional and complementary therapies, such as **doctors**, **naturopaths**, **chiropractors**, **acupuncturists**, and **nutritionists**, to create a treatment plan that works for the patient as a whole.

A key component of integrative care is **preventive health**. Unlike traditional medicine, which often focuses on treating diseases after they occur, integrative care places a strong emphasis on preventing illness before it begins. This proactive approach might include lifestyle modifications such as dietary changes, stress reduction techniques, exercise programs, and emotional wellness practices. Preventive care in an integrative framework often involves **nutrition therapy, herbal medicine, mindfulness practices**, and **detoxification** programs aimed at boosting the body's natural defenses and optimizing its health.

Another significant aspect of integrative care is the use of **mind-body therapies**, which recognize the powerful connection between mental, emotional, and physical health. Practices like **meditation, yoga, guided imagery**, and **breathing exercises** are often incorporated to reduce stress, improve emotional resilience, and promote mental clarity. These techniques are supported by evidence showing that managing stress and improving emotional health can have significant physical health benefits, such as improved immune function, reduced inflammation, and better cardiovascular health.

Pain management is one area where integrative care has demonstrated significant effectiveness. Chronic pain, whether from conditions like **arthritis, fibromyalgia, headaches**, or **back pain**, can be debilitating. Integrative care provides patients with a wide array of treatment options, including **acupuncture, chiropractic adjustments, massage therapy**, and **herbal remedies** in addition to conventional pain medications. These alternative therapies often complement pharmaceutical treatments, reducing the need for painkillers, minimizing side effects, and improving quality of life.

Chronic disease management also falls within the scope of integrative care. Conditions like **diabetes, heart disease, autoimmune disorders**, and **obesity** require long-term management, and integrative care offers a comprehensive approach. Conventional treatments, such as medications or surgical interventions, are paired with dietary changes, physical activity, stress management, and emotional support. For example, someone with heart disease may receive medication and undergo surgery if needed, but they may also be encouraged to adopt a heart-healthy diet, incorporate stress-relieving practices like meditation, and engage in physical activity tailored to their abilities. This integrated approach helps address the root causes of chronic conditions, reduces complications, and improves overall health.

Cancer care is another area where integrative medicine has been widely used, helping patients manage the physical and emotional burdens of the disease and its treatment. Integrative care offers supportive therapies such as **acupuncture** for pain relief, **aromatherapy** to reduce anxiety, and **nutritional counseling** to support the immune system during chemotherapy. These therapies are used alongside conventional cancer treatments like chemotherapy, radiation, and surgery to improve quality of life, reduce side effects, and support recovery. Many integrative care centers now work directly with oncology teams to ensure that complementary therapies do not interfere with conventional treatments but instead provide additional benefits to the patient's healing process.

Women's health is also a field where integrative care can be particularly effective. Conditions such as **menstrual disorders**, **fertility challenges**, **pregnancy support**, and **menopause symptoms** can be addressed through both conventional treatments and alternative therapies. For example, women experiencing **menopause** may use hormonal therapy in conjunction with acupuncture, herbal remedies, or lifestyle adjustments to manage symptoms like hot flashes, mood swings, and sleep disturbances. **Fertility treatments** may be complemented with acupuncture, nutritional counseling, or stress management techniques to enhance the chances of conception and support overall reproductive health.

In **mental health care**, integrative treatments are often used alongside traditional psychiatric medications to help patients manage conditions like **anxiety, depression, post-traumatic stress disorder (PTSD)**, and **insomnia**. Integrative practitioners may recommend a combination of **talk therapy, mindfulness practices, herbal supplements, yoga**, and **exercise** to address both the symptoms and underlying causes of mental health conditions. These therapies can work in synergy with conventional medications, helping to alleviate symptoms more effectively and reduce reliance on pharmaceuticals over time.

In conclusion, the scope of integrative care is vast, encompassing a wide range of therapies and practices that address the whole person. From preventive health and chronic disease management to pain relief, mental health support, and cancer care, integrative medicine provides a comprehensive approach to healing. By combining the best of conventional and alternative medicine, integrative care offers a personalized and holistic path to health that recognizes the interconnectedness of body, mind, and spirit. This approach not only focuses on treating illness but also on enhancing overall well-being and preventing future health problems, empowering patients to take an active role in their own healing process.

Integrative Medicine Case Studies

Integrative medicine blends conventional medical treatments with complementary therapies to treat the whole person—body, mind, and spirit. This approach is often used for managing chronic conditions, improving overall well-being, and supporting healing during and after illness. Case studies from integrative medicine practices illustrate the potential benefits of combining conventional and alternative therapies to enhance patient outcomes and improve quality of life.

One case study involves a patient with **chronic pain** due to **fibromyalgia**, a condition characterized by widespread pain, fatigue, and tenderness in muscles and joints. Traditional medical treatments, such as pain medication and anti-inflammatory drugs, provided limited relief. The patient, under the care of an integrative medicine specialist, was given a treatment plan that included **acupuncture, nutritional therapy**, and **mindfulness-based stress reduction (MBSR)**. Acupuncture was used to stimulate specific points on the body to reduce pain and improve energy flow, while the nutritional plan focused on anti-inflammatory foods and supplements like **omega-3 fatty acids** to reduce inflammation. MBSR sessions helped the patient manage the emotional and psychological aspects of chronic pain, such as stress and anxiety. Over time, the patient reported a significant reduction in pain, improved sleep, and better overall energy levels. This case highlights how integrative medicine can provide a more holistic approach to managing chronic conditions that may not fully respond to conventional treatments alone.

In another case, an individual diagnosed with **breast cancer** sought integrative care to complement their conventional cancer treatments. The patient was undergoing chemotherapy and radiation therapy, which were causing debilitating side effects such as nausea, fatigue, and loss of appetite. In addition to conventional treatments, the patient worked with an integrative team that included a nutritionist, acupuncturist, and massage therapist. The nutritionist recommended a diet rich in **antioxidants** and **anti-inflammatory foods**, such as berries, leafy greens, and turmeric, to support the immune system and reduce inflammation. Acupuncture sessions helped alleviate nausea and pain, while massage therapy provided relief from muscle tension and promoted relaxation. The integrative care team also provided emotional support through mindfulness practices and stress management techniques, helping the patient cope with the emotional burden of cancer. The patient experienced fewer side effects from chemotherapy, improved mood, and better quality of life during treatment. This case underscores how integrative therapies can support the body's healing process and mitigate the side effects of conventional cancer treatments.

Another compelling case study involves a patient with **irritable bowel syndrome (IBS)**, a digestive disorder that causes symptoms like abdominal pain, bloating, and changes in bowel movements. The patient had been treated with prescription medications for several years, but the symptoms persisted, and side effects from the medication began to affect quality of life. The integrative approach included **dietary modifications**, **probiotics**, **acupuncture**, and **stress reduction techniques**. The nutritionist advised a **low-FODMAP diet**, which is designed to reduce symptoms by eliminating certain fermentable carbohydrates that can trigger IBS symptoms.

Probiotic supplements were introduced to promote gut health and restore balance to the digestive system. Acupuncture was used to address digestive disturbances and manage stress, as anxiety is often linked to IBS flare-ups. Over the course of several months, the patient experienced a significant improvement in digestion, reduced bloating, and fewer episodes of pain. This case illustrates how integrative medicine can effectively manage chronic conditions like IBS by addressing underlying factors such as diet, gut health, and stress.

In a case involving **chronic stress** and **anxiety**, an integrative approach helped a patient who was experiencing persistent anxiety symptoms that were not fully controlled with medication alone. The patient had been prescribed **antidepressants** and **anxiolytics**, but still struggled with emotional regulation, sleep disturbances, and a heightened stress response. The integrative team introduced **mind-body techniques**, such as **yoga, breathing exercises**, and **cognitive-behavioral therapy (CBT)**, in combination with continued medication management. The yoga sessions focused on **relaxation, breath control**, and **mindfulness**, helping the patient become more aware of their body and emotions. Breathing exercises, such as **diaphragmatic breathing** and **pranayama**, helped calm the nervous system and reduce anxiety in stressful situations. CBT was used to address thought patterns and behaviors that contributed to the patient's anxiety. Over time, the patient reported a reduction in anxiety symptoms, improved sleep, and a greater sense of emotional balance. This case highlights how integrative medicine can support mental health by addressing both the psychological and physiological components of anxiety.

A final case involves a patient with **chronic fatigue syndrome (CFS)**, a condition characterized by extreme fatigue that doesn't improve with rest and is often accompanied by sleep disturbances, memory issues, and muscle pain. After extensive testing and treatment with conventional medicine, the patient found little relief. The integrative approach included **nutritional therapy, acupuncture,** and **mindfulness practices**. The nutritionist recommended a personalized diet to support mitochondrial function, increase energy levels, and address potential nutritional deficiencies. Acupuncture was used to stimulate energy flow and alleviate fatigue, while mindfulness and relaxation techniques helped manage the psychological stress often associated with chronic fatigue. Over several months, the patient reported significant improvements in energy, sleep quality, and mental clarity. This case demonstrates how integrative medicine can offer a multifaceted approach to managing complex and poorly understood conditions like chronic fatigue syndrome.

In conclusion, integrative medicine offers a powerful and personalized approach to healthcare by combining the strengths of both conventional and alternative therapies. Case studies show how this approach can provide comprehensive care that addresses not only physical symptoms but also emotional and mental well-being. By integrating diffcrcnt healing modalities—such as acupuncture, nutrition therapy, yoga, and mind-body techniques—patients can experience improved outcomes, better quality of life, and a more holistic path to healing. Integrative medicine highlights the value of personalized care, collaboration among healthcare providers, and treating the whole person, offering a promising approach to managing both chronic and acute health conditions.

Research and Studies on Alternative Medicine

Research into alternative medicine has been steadily growing over the past few decades as more people seek natural, non-pharmaceutical treatments for a variety of health conditions. While the body of scientific evidence supporting alternative therapies is still evolving, many studies have highlighted the potential benefits of practices like **acupuncture, herbal medicine, mind-body therapies**, and **chiropractic care**. These treatments, often used in conjunction with conventional medical practices, aim to address the root causes of illness and promote holistic well-being.

One of the most well-researched forms of alternative medicine is **acupuncture**. Numerous studies have shown its effectiveness in managing **chronic pain** conditions, including **back pain, osteoarthritis**, and **headaches**. A 2012 meta-analysis published in the *Archives of Internal Medicine* analyzed over 17,000 patients and found that acupuncture was more effective than placebo treatments for chronic pain. Acupuncture is thought to work by stimulating the body's nervous system, which may enhance the release of endorphins and other neurochemicals that reduce pain and inflammation. Additionally, acupuncture is used for conditions such as **stress, insomnia**, and **digestive disorders**, and research into its broader therapeutic effects continues to grow.

Herbal medicine has long been used as a form of alternative therapy, with plants like **turmeric, ginger, echinacea**, and **ginseng** frequently recommended for their medicinal properties. A growing body of evidence supports the use of herbal remedies in treating a variety of ailments. For instance, **turmeric** and its active compound **curcumin** have been extensively researched for their anti-inflammatory and antioxidant properties. Studies suggest that curcumin may play a role in reducing the symptoms of inflammatory conditions like **rheumatoid arthritis** and **ulcerative colitis**. Additionally, **ginseng** has been shown to improve energy levels, reduce fatigue, and enhance cognitive function, particularly in people with **chronic fatigue syndrome** and **stress-related conditions**. However, while many studies demonstrate promising results, the quality and consistency of research in herbal medicine can vary, and it's important to approach herbal remedies with caution, as some may interact with prescription medications.

Mind-body therapies, including **meditation, yoga, hypnotherapy**, and **mindfulness-based stress reduction (MBSR),** have been increasingly studied for their impact on mental and physical health. For example, MBSR, which involves mindfulness meditation and body awareness techniques, has been shown to reduce symptoms of **anxiety, depression**, and **chronic pain**. A 2016 study in the *Journal of Clinical Psychology* found that MBSR was as effective as traditional cognitive behavioral therapy (CBT) in treating anxiety and depression in patients with **generalized anxiety disorder**. Similarly, yoga, with its combination of physical postures, breathing exercises, and meditation, has been found to improve flexibility, reduce stress, and help manage chronic conditions such as **hypertension** and **type 2 diabetes**. Research into these therapies shows that they have significant potential for improving overall well-being, especially when combined with other forms of treatment.

In **chiropractic care**, the focus is on spinal health and musculoskeletal disorders. Chiropractors use manual manipulation techniques to adjust misalignments in the spine, with the goal of improving nerve function and relieving pain. Numerous studies support the use of chiropractic treatments for **lower back pain**, **neck pain**, and **headaches**. A 2018 study published in the *Journal of the American Medical Association* concluded that spinal manipulation was effective in treating acute lower back pain, and the American College of Physicians has recommended spinal manipulation as part of a comprehensive approach to pain management. Chiropractors often collaborate with other healthcare providers to manage complex conditions and are an important part of the integrative medicine model.

Homeopathy remains one of the most debated alternative medicine practices. Homeopathy is based on the idea that substances that cause symptoms in a healthy person can, in very diluted forms, treat similar symptoms in a sick person. Despite its widespread use, homeopathy has faced significant skepticism in the scientific community. Several studies have failed to show that homeopathic treatments are more effective than placebos. However, some studies suggest that the placebo effect may play a significant role in homeopathy's perceived benefits, particularly in conditions like **chronic pain**, **insomnia**, and **irritable bowel syndrome**. While the scientific support for homeopathy remains limited, it continues to be a popular treatment for those seeking non-invasive, natural remedies.

Energy medicine, which includes practices such as **Reiki**, **Healing Touch**, and **therapeutic touch**, is an emerging field in alternative medicine. These therapies are based on the idea that the body has a field of energy that can be manipulated to promote healing. Research in this area is still in its early stages, but some studies suggest that energy therapies may help reduce pain, anxiety, and stress. For instance, a 2010 study published in *The Journal of Alternative and Complementary Medicine* found that Reiki was effective in reducing pain and anxiety in patients undergoing surgery. While more rigorous studies are needed, early findings indicate that energy-based therapies can complement conventional treatments by promoting relaxation and supporting the body's natural healing processes.

One area where alternative medicine has garnered increasing attention is in the **management of chronic disease**. **Integrative medicine** combines conventional treatments with alternative therapies to provide a more comprehensive approach to chronic illnesses such as **cancer, diabetes**, and **heart disease**. Case studies show that patients who combine conventional treatments with therapies like **acupuncture, nutrition counseling, herbal supplements**, and **stress management** techniques often experience better outcomes, including improved quality of life and reduced side effects. Research on integrative care supports the idea that a combination of conventional and alternative approaches can optimize patient health, particularly in managing chronic conditions that require long-term care.

In conclusion, research into alternative medicine continues to expand, with promising findings in areas such as acupuncture, herbal medicine, mind-body therapies, chiropractic care, and energy healing. While more research is needed to fully understand the mechanisms behind many of these therapies, the growing body of evidence indicates that alternative medicine can play an important role in health and wellness. Many people are seeking holistic, non-invasive treatments to complement conventional medicine, and continued research will help clarify how these therapies can be integrated into modern healthcare to improve patient outcomes.

Overview of Studies

Studies on alternative medicine have steadily increased as more individuals seek natural, non-pharmaceutical approaches to health and wellness. These studies examine the effectiveness, safety, and mechanisms of alternative therapies such as **acupuncture, herbal medicine, chiropractic care, energy healing**, and **mind-body therapies**. While much of the research is still ongoing and evolving, the growing body of evidence suggests that many alternative therapies can offer valuable benefits when used alongside or in place of conventional treatments.

One area of alternative medicine that has received significant attention in recent years is **acupuncture**. Numerous studies have investigated its efficacy in treating a variety of conditions, particularly **chronic pain**. For example, a 2012 meta-analysis published in the *Archives of Internal Medicine* reviewed more than 17,000 patients and found that acupuncture was significantly more effective than placebo treatments in managing chronic pain, including **back pain, osteoarthritis**, and **headaches**. This research suggests that acupuncture may stimulate the release of natural painkillers, such as **endorphins**, and influence areas of the brain associated with pain processing. Despite these findings, more rigorous studies are still needed to fully understand how acupuncture works and its long-term effects.

In **herbal medicine**, various plant-based remedies have been the subject of scientific inquiry, with many studies supporting their therapeutic benefits. **Turmeric**, for instance, contains the active compound **curcumin**, known for its anti-inflammatory and antioxidant properties. Research has shown that turmeric may help reduce inflammation in conditions like **rheumatoid arthritis, irritable bowel syndrome**, and **osteoarthritis**. Similarly, **ginseng**, a widely used adaptogen, has been studied for its ability to improve energy levels and reduce fatigue, especially in patients with **chronic fatigue syndrome** or those recovering from illness. However, while these herbal remedies show promise, not all studies have reached conclusive results, and more research is necessary to establish standardized dosages and long-term effects.

Chiropractic care, focusing on spinal adjustments and musculoskeletal health, has been the subject of numerous studies examining its effectiveness in treating **lower back pain**, **neck pain**, and **headaches**. The *Journal of the American Medical Association* published a study in 2017 that found spinal manipulation to be an effective treatment for acute lower back pain. Chiropractors often use manual spinal adjustments to improve mobility, reduce pain, and promote nerve function, and research suggests that this technique is particularly beneficial for musculoskeletal disorders. Chiropractic care is increasingly being integrated into broader health management strategies, especially for patients with chronic pain who seek non-invasive alternatives to medication.

Mind-body therapies, such as **meditation, yoga**, and **mindfulness-based stress reduction (MBSR)**, have been the subject of numerous studies exploring their impact on mental and physical health. Research has shown that mindfulness meditation can significantly reduce symptoms of **anxiety**, **depression**, and **chronic pain**. A 2016 study published in the *Journal of Clinical Psychology* demonstrated that MBSR was as effective as cognitive-behavioral therapy (CBT) in treating anxiety. Yoga, which combines physical postures with controlled breathing and mindfulness, has been found to improve flexibility, reduce stress, and aid in managing conditions like **hypertension** and **diabetes**. Many studies suggest that these mind-body practices can help improve overall mental well-being, reduce stress hormones, and promote relaxation, offering a holistic approach to emotional health.

In the realm of **energy medicine**, research is still in its early stages, but there is growing interest in therapies like **Reiki** and **therapeutic touch**. These therapies involve the transfer of energy from a practitioner to a patient to promote healing and balance. Several studies have explored the effects of Reiki on **pain management**, **anxiety**, and **stress reduction**. For instance, a 2010 study published in *The Journal of Alternative and Complementary Medicine* found that Reiki significantly reduced pain and anxiety in patients undergoing surgery. Although scientific consensus is still lacking on the mechanisms behind energy healing, these early findings suggest that these therapies may have positive effects on mental and physical health, especially in terms of relaxation and stress relief.

Homeopathy, one of the most controversial areas of alternative medicine, continues to be debated in the scientific community. Homeopathy is based on the principle that a substance that causes symptoms in a healthy person can, when diluted, treat those same symptoms in a sick person. While there is a large body of anecdotal evidence supporting homeopathy's effectiveness in treating a wide range of conditions, many studies have failed to show that homeopathic remedies are more effective than placebos. A 2009 study published in *The Lancet* found little evidence to support the use of homeopathy beyond the placebo effect. Despite this, homeopathy remains a popular alternative therapy, with ongoing research exploring its potential mechanisms and therapeutic uses.

Integrative medicine, which combines conventional treatments with alternative therapies, is another area where research is expanding. Studies on integrative medicine suggest that combining approaches like acupuncture, massage, herbal supplements, and mind-body therapies with conventional treatments can improve patient outcomes, particularly for chronic conditions such as **cancer**, **heart disease**, and **diabetes**. For example, a study on cancer patients found that acupuncture and massage significantly reduced chemotherapy-induced nausea, pain, and fatigue. Integrative medicine offers a promising model for patients who wish to receive comprehensive care that addresses both physical symptoms and emotional well-being.

In conclusion, research into alternative medicine is a rapidly expanding field with a growing body of evidence supporting the effectiveness of many therapies. Practices such as acupuncture, herbal medicine, chiropractic care, and mind-body therapies are becoming increasingly recognized for their ability to treat a wide variety of health conditions, particularly when combined with conventional treatments. While there are still gaps in scientific understanding, ongoing studies continue to shed light on the potential benefits of alternative medicine, offering more comprehensive treatment options for those seeking holistic, non-invasive therapies.

Scientifically-Backed Benefits

Alternative medicine encompasses a wide range of therapies, many of which have been the subject of scientific studies that validate their effectiveness in treating various health conditions. From **acupuncture** and **herbal medicine** to **mind-body practices** and **chiropractic care**, scientific research has provided evidence to support the benefits of these treatments. While alternative therapies are often used in conjunction with conventional medicine, their scientifically-backed benefits demonstrate that they can be effective in improving health and well-being across different domains.

One of the most widely studied alternative treatments is **acupuncture**, which involves the insertion of thin needles into specific points on the body to stimulate energy flow and restore balance. Scientific studies have shown that acupuncture can be highly effective in managing **chronic pain** conditions, such as **back pain, osteoarthritis, migraine headaches**, and **fibromyalgia**. A meta-analysis published in *The Archives of Internal Medicine* in 2012 reviewed 17,000 patients and found that acupuncture was significantly more effective than a placebo in treating chronic pain. Acupuncture has also been shown to improve circulation, reduce inflammation, and promote the release of pain-relieving chemicals like endorphins. This evidence underscores acupuncture's ability to address both physical pain and overall well-being.

Herbal medicine is another area where scientific research has demonstrated the effectiveness of alternative treatments. Plants such as **turmeric, ginger**, and **echinacea** have been studied for their therapeutic properties. **Curcumin,** the active compound in turmeric, is well-known for its **anti-inflammatory** and **antioxidant** effects. Research has shown that curcumin can reduce inflammation and may be beneficial in conditions such as **rheumatoid arthritis, osteoarthritis,** and **ulcerative colitis**. Similarly, **ginger** has been shown to alleviate **nausea**, especially in patients undergoing chemotherapy, and can help reduce muscle pain and inflammation. **Echinacea**, commonly used to boost the immune system, has been studied for its ability to reduce the duration and severity of **common colds**. Although not all herbal treatments have been subjected to extensive clinical trials, those that have been researched provide strong evidence of their efficacy in supporting health and managing conditions naturally.

Mind-body therapies—which include **meditation**, **yoga**, and **mindfulness-based stress reduction (MBSR)**—have gained increasing recognition for their scientifically-backed benefits. A growing body of research indicates that these practices can significantly reduce symptoms of **anxiety**, **depression**, and **chronic pain**. Studies have shown that **mindfulness meditation** can alter brain activity, enhancing areas responsible for emotional regulation and reducing areas linked to stress. A 2016 study in the *Journal of Clinical Psychology* found that mindfulness meditation was as effective as cognitive-behavioral therapy (CBT) in treating **generalized anxiety disorder**. **Yoga** has been found to improve flexibility, reduce stress, and enhance overall physical and mental health. A systematic review in the *Journal of Clinical Psychology* concluded that yoga-based interventions significantly improved mental health outcomes, particularly in those dealing with **depression** and **anxiety**. These mind-body practices are now widely recommended by healthcare providers as a complementary treatment for managing stress, improving mood, and enhancing overall wellness.

Chiropractic care, which focuses on the manipulation and adjustment of the spine, is another area where scientific evidence supports its effectiveness. Numerous studies have found that chiropractic adjustments can be effective in treating **lower back pain, neck pain**, and **headaches**. A study published in the *Journal of the American Medical Association* in 2017 found that spinal manipulation was an effective treatment for acute lower back pain. Chiropractic care has also been shown to improve range of motion, reduce muscle stiffness, and support better posture. While chiropractic adjustments are most commonly used for musculoskeletal pain, they can also be part of a broader approach to overall health, including improved sleep and stress relief.

Massage therapy is another alternative treatment that has been widely studied for its scientifically supported benefits. Research has shown that massage can effectively reduce **muscle tension**, alleviate **chronic pain**, and reduce **stress**. A 2010 study published in the *Journal of Alternative and Complementary Medicine* found that therapeutic massage helped reduce **anxiety, muscle soreness**, and **pain** in patients suffering from various conditions, including **fibromyalgia** and **arthritis**. Massage therapy has also been shown to improve circulation, support lymphatic drainage, and promote relaxation by lowering **cortisol** levels (the stress hormone) and increasing **serotonin** and **dopamine**, which are associated with positive mood regulation.

Aromatherapy, which uses essential oils for therapeutic purposes, has been supported by research showing its effectiveness in treating conditions like **stress, insomnia**, and **mood disorders**. Essential oils such as **lavender** have been shown to reduce anxiety and promote relaxation, while

peppermint oil can help alleviate headaches and improve focus. A study published in *The International Journal of Neuroscience* found that inhaling lavender essential oil significantly reduced anxiety and promoted a calming effect in participants. Aromatherapy is increasingly being used in hospitals and wellness centers to help patients manage stress, anxiety, and even post-surgical recovery.

In **energy medicine**, therapies like **Reiki** and **therapeutic touch** are gaining attention for their potential to promote relaxation and pain relief. Though scientific research on energy medicine is still in its early stages, several studies suggest that these therapies can help reduce **pain**, **stress**, and **anxiety**. A 2010 study in the *Journal of Alternative and Complementary Medicine* found that Reiki significantly reduced pain and anxiety in patients undergoing surgery. These therapies are believed to work by promoting a sense of calm and facilitating the body's natural healing mechanisms.

In conclusion, alternative medicine offers a wide range of therapies that are supported by scientific research for their effectiveness in managing and treating various health conditions. From acupuncture's success in pain management to the mind-body benefits of yoga and meditation, scientific evidence continues to affirm the role of alternative therapies in promoting health and wellness. While ongoing research is necessary to further explore the mechanisms behind these treatments, many alternative therapies are already recognized for their ability to complement conventional medicine, reduce symptoms, and enhance overall quality of life.

Current Research in the Field

Current research in the field of alternative medicine is rapidly expanding as scientists, healthcare professionals, and patients alike explore the potential benefits of complementary therapies in managing health conditions. This research is focused on validating the effectiveness of treatments such as **acupuncture**, **herbal medicine**, **mind-body practices**, **chiropractic care**, and **energy healing**, as well as understanding the mechanisms behind these therapies. While there are still gaps in knowledge, recent studies suggest that alternative medicine can play a valuable role in improving health outcomes and enhancing the quality of life.

One area of active research is the use of **acupuncture** for pain management and chronic conditions. A growing body of evidence supports its effectiveness in treating various types of pain, including **back pain**, **osteoarthritis**, **headaches**, and **fibromyalgia**. A 2020 systematic review and meta-analysis published in *JAMA Network Open* examined data from over 20,000 patients and found that acupuncture was significantly more effective than placebo in reducing pain and improving physical function in individuals with chronic pain. Studies are also investigating acupuncture's potential to improve conditions like **anxiety** and **insomnia**, and its effects on the **nervous system** and **circulatory health**. Research in this area continues to explore the precise biological mechanisms through which acupuncture affects pain pathways and promotes healing.

Herbal medicine remains one of the most widely used forms of alternative therapy, and its application is being increasingly examined in clinical research. Plants like **turmeric**, **ginger**, **echinacea**, and **ginseng** are among the most researched herbs due to their anti-inflammatory, immune-boosting, and adaptogenic properties. For instance, **turmeric** and its active ingredient, **curcumin**, are being studied for their ability to treat **inflammatory diseases**, such as **arthritis** and **ulcerative colitis**. A study published in *Phytotherapy Research* in 2020 found that curcumin supplementation helped reduce symptoms of **osteoarthritis** by improving joint function and decreasing inflammation. Research on **ginseng** continues to explore its potential in improving energy levels, cognitive function, and stress resilience, particularly in people with **chronic fatigue syndrome** and **adrenal fatigue**.

Another active area of study involves **mind-body therapies**, such as **meditation, yoga**, and **mindfulness-based stress reduction (MBSR)**. These practices have long been recognized for their ability to reduce stress and improve mental health, but recent research is expanding into their effects on physical health as well. Studies have shown that **meditation** can reduce **blood pressure**, improve **heart rate variability**, and help manage conditions like **anxiety, depression**, and **chronic pain**. A 2018 study in *JAMA Internal Medicine* found that mindfulness meditation was associated with reduced levels of **cortisol** (a stress hormone) and enhanced immune function. **Yoga** has also been shown to improve flexibility, strength, and mobility, particularly in patients with **arthritis** or **back pain**. Additionally, ongoing research continues to investigate the long-term benefits of these therapies, particularly their ability to reduce inflammation, lower the risk of chronic diseases, and improve overall health outcomes.

Chiropractic care is another field that is experiencing growth in research, particularly regarding the treatment of musculoskeletal pain. Recent studies have confirmed the efficacy of chiropractic spinal manipulation in treating **lower back pain**, **neck pain**, and **headaches**. A 2017 study published in *The Lancet* found that spinal manipulation was as effective as other treatments, including physical therapy and medication, in managing acute low back pain. Chiropractic care is also being explored for its role in enhancing general **wellness**, including its effects on **immune function**, **sleep quality**, and stress reduction. Ongoing research is focusing on understanding how spinal adjustments influence nervous system function and contribute to overall health.

Energy healing practices, such as **Reiki** and **therapeutic touch**, are gaining attention in both clinical and scientific communities. These therapies involve manipulating the energy fields around the body to promote healing and restore balance. While there is still skepticism about how energy healing works, several studies suggest that it can have positive effects on **stress**, **anxiety**, **pain relief**, and **wound healing**. For example, a 2021 study published in *The Journal of Alternative and Complementary Medicine* showed that Reiki therapy significantly reduced pain and anxiety in patients undergoing surgery. Research is currently investigating the physiological mechanisms behind energy healing, including how it might influence the **autonomic nervous system**, **cortisol levels**, and **endocrine function**.

Integrative medicine, which combines conventional treatments with alternative therapies, continues to be a key area of research. Studies are increasingly focusing on how integrative approaches can improve the management of **chronic diseases** such as **cancer**, **diabetes**, and **heart disease**. For example, patients undergoing **cancer treatments** such as chemotherapy have reported improved quality of life and fewer side effects when acupuncture, **massage therapy**, and **mindfulness** are used alongside conventional care. Research suggests that integrative medicine not only alleviates physical symptoms but also supports emotional well-being, reduces stress, and improves treatment outcomes. The growing body of evidence highlights the potential of combining conventional medical care with alternative therapies to optimize healing and enhance patient satisfaction.

In conclusion, current research in alternative medicine continues to expand and provide valuable insights into the effectiveness of treatments like acupuncture, herbal medicine, chiropractic care, and mind-body therapies. While many areas of alternative medicine still require more rigorous scientific investigation, existing studies offer strong evidence for the benefits of these therapies in managing pain, improving mental health, and promoting overall wellness. As more research is conducted, the integration of alternative medicine into conventional healthcare systems may become increasingly common, offering patients a comprehensive approach to health that addresses both physical and emotional well-being.

Risks and Challenges of Alternative Medicine

While alternative medicine offers a variety of benefits, there are also inherent risks and challenges that need to be considered. These risks can range from **ineffectiveness** to **adverse reactions**, and they underscore the importance of a balanced approach when considering alternative therapies. Understanding these potential risks can help individuals make informed decisions about integrating alternative medicine into their healthcare routines.

One of the primary risks associated with alternative medicine is the **lack of scientific evidence** for certain therapies. While some alternative treatments, like acupuncture or certain herbal remedies, have been well-studied and supported by research, many other practices lack substantial clinical evidence to confirm their effectiveness. For example, while **homeopathy** is widely used for various conditions, there is little empirical evidence to support its efficacy beyond the placebo effect. Similarly, some alternative therapies are based on traditional practices without rigorous testing or validation in modern scientific research, making it difficult for patients to know whether the treatment will be effective or safe.

Adverse reactions and side effects are another significant concern with alternative medicine. Natural does not always mean safe, and certain herbal remedies or treatments may interact with prescription medications or cause allergic reactions. For instance, herbs like **St. John's Wort**, often used for depression, can interfere with antidepressant medications, birth control pills, and anticoagulants, leading to unwanted side effects or reduced effectiveness of conventional drugs. **Ginseng** has been known to cause headaches, sleep disturbances, and high blood pressure in some individuals. **Echinacea**, frequently used to boost the immune system, can lead to allergic reactions in those who are allergic to plants in the daisy family. It is essential for individuals using alternative therapies to consult with a healthcare provider to ensure that they do not experience harmful interactions with other treatments or conditions.

Delayed treatment is another risk of relying solely on alternative medicine. In some cases, individuals may turn to alternative therapies when they are not receiving adequate results from conventional treatments, or they may use alternative medicine in lieu of conventional care for serious conditions. For instance, relying on **herbal treatments** or **energy healing** for conditions like cancer, diabetes, or heart disease instead of seeking proper medical care can delay the diagnosis and treatment of life-threatening diseases. The risks of forgoing conventional medical treatments in favor of unproven alternative therapies can be particularly severe for serious health conditions, as these therapies may not be sufficient to manage or cure the underlying issue.

There is also the issue of **quality control** and **regulation** within the field of alternative medicine. Unlike conventional drugs, which are tightly regulated by agencies such as the **Food and Drug Administration (FDA)**, many alternative therapies, particularly **herbal supplements**, are not subject to the same rigorous standards. This lack of regulation can lead to inconsistencies in quality, potency, and purity. Some herbal supplements may contain contaminants, such as **heavy metals**, **pesticides**, or other toxins, which could pose health risks. A study published in *JAMA Internal Medicine* in 2013 found that 59% of herbal products contained ingredients not listed on the label, raising concerns about the safety and transparency of these products.

Another challenge is the **training and qualifications** of alternative medicine practitioners. The training required to practice alternative therapies varies greatly depending on the treatment and location, and some practitioners may not be licensed or adequately trained. For example, while licensed acupuncturists are required to undergo specific training, there are few standardized educational requirements for those offering complementary therapies like energy healing or **aromatherapy**. This variability in qualifications can affect the quality of care and increase the risk of harm or improper treatment.

Additionally, there is a **psychological risk** involved with alternative medicine, particularly in areas where patients may feel misled or disappointed by the outcomes of treatment. The use of alternative therapies is often accompanied by high patient expectations, and when these treatments fail to deliver the desired results, it can lead to **emotional distress** and **disillusionment**. This is particularly concerning for patients who have invested significant time, money, and hope into therapies that do not live up to their promises. This psychological burden can further complicate the patient's overall well-being, particularly if they are simultaneously dealing with chronic illness or pain.

The **cost** of alternative treatments is another barrier that can impact their accessibility and benefit. Many alternative therapies, such as **chiropractic care**, **acupuncture**, and **herbal supplements**, are not always covered by health insurance plans, making them financially burdensome for some individuals. Additionally, the need for ongoing treatments or long-term use of supplements can further drive up costs. For patients without sufficient insurance coverage, these financial barriers may make it difficult to access necessary care, potentially leaving them in a situation where they rely on therapies that are not effective, rather than seeking conventional care that might address their medical needs more directly.

Lastly, the **lack of standardization** in alternative medicine presents challenges in both patient care and scientific research. Since many alternative practices are based on traditional or holistic principles, the treatments and dosages may vary widely between practitioners, making it difficult to measure effectiveness or establish treatment protocols. This inconsistency also makes it harder to conduct large-scale clinical trials or create standardized guidelines for practitioners. Without consistent practices, patients may experience varying levels of care or benefit from treatment, depending on the practitioner's experience and approach.

In conclusion, while alternative medicine offers many potential benefits, it also comes with significant risks and challenges. The lack of scientific evidence for some therapies, the possibility of adverse interactions with conventional medications, delayed treatment for serious conditions, and variability in the quality and regulation of treatments all pose potential hazards. It is crucial for patients to be well-informed, seek guidance from qualified practitioners, and collaborate with their healthcare providers to ensure that any alternative treatments they pursue are safe, appropriate, and effective. Combining the best of both conventional and alternative medicine can provide a comprehensive and balanced approach to health, but it requires careful consideration and oversight.

Understanding the Risks

When considering alternative medicine, it's essential to understand the potential risks involved. While many people seek out complementary therapies for their natural healing properties, these treatments are not without their challenges. From **unproven effectiveness** to **adverse reactions** and **interactions** with other medications, the risks of alternative medicine should not be overlooked. Understanding these risks allows individuals to make informed decisions and use alternative therapies safely alongside conventional treatments.

One of the primary risks of alternative medicine is the **lack of scientific evidence** for many therapies. While some practices, like **acupuncture** and **herbal medicine**, have been studied extensively and have demonstrated benefits, many others have not undergone the same rigorous clinical testing. Without substantial scientific support, it can be difficult to determine the true effectiveness of certain alternative treatments. For example, **homeopathy**, which relies on highly diluted substances, has been widely criticized for lacking empirical evidence of its therapeutic effects. The absence of scientific backing raises concerns about whether these treatments are genuinely beneficial or simply placebos.

Adverse reactions are another critical risk, especially when patients use alternative medicine in conjunction with conventional medications. **Herbal remedies** can cause allergic reactions or side effects, especially when they are not properly dosed or when they interact with other medications. For instance, **St. John's Wort**, commonly used for depression, can interfere with antidepressants, birth control pills, and anticoagulants, leading to dangerous complications. **Ginseng**, often used to combat fatigue, can increase blood pressure or cause insomnia in some people. As many alternative remedies are not subject to the same regulatory standards as pharmaceuticals, there is also the risk of **contaminants** like **heavy metals**, **pesticides**, or **adulterants** in some herbal products, which can harm the body rather than help it.

Delayed diagnosis and treatment is another concern when relying solely on alternative medicine. While complementary therapies can be helpful, they should not replace conventional treatments, especially for serious or life-threatening conditions. For example, someone with **cancer** might choose to pursue herbal or alternative treatments while forgoing conventional medical care like chemotherapy or radiation. This delay in receiving appropriate treatment could allow the condition to worsen, ultimately reducing the chances of successful recovery. Many alternative therapies are not designed to treat serious diseases and may only address symptoms rather than the root cause of the illness.

There is also the risk of **misleading information**. Because the field of alternative medicine is not as strictly regulated as conventional healthcare, consumers may be exposed to unqualified practitioners who promote unproven treatments or exaggerated claims. This can lead to false hope or financial loss for patients seeking relief from chronic conditions. For example, some practitioners may promise quick cures for chronic illnesses like **arthritis** or **diabetes**, even though the treatment may have little scientific merit. This can create an environment where patients feel pressured into expensive treatments that offer little to no benefit, undermining their trust in both alternative and conventional medical care.

The **lack of standardization** in alternative medicine can also pose significant risks. Many alternative therapies lack established guidelines or protocols, which can lead to inconsistent treatment and outcomes. For instance, dosages of **herbal supplements** can vary widely depending on the manufacturer, leading to variations in potency and safety. Furthermore, some treatments, such as **energy healing** or **chiropractic adjustments**, may not be practiced consistently from one practitioner to another. This lack of standardization means that results can vary significantly, and patients may not always receive the same level of care or benefit from therapy, even when using the same treatment method.

Another concern is the **psychological impact** that certain alternative treatments can have. Patients may develop a strong belief in the healing power of a specific therapy and, when it fails to provide the expected results, may experience feelings of disappointment, frustration, or distress. This can be particularly problematic for individuals who may already be struggling with a serious health issue, as it can exacerbate feelings of helplessness or depression. Additionally, a focus on alternative therapies can sometimes lead patients to neglect the psychological and emotional aspects of their illness, such as **anxiety** or **stress**, which can impact recovery and overall health.

Lastly, the **cost** of alternative therapies can be a significant barrier. Many alternative treatments, such as **chiropractic care**, **acupuncture**, and **herbal supplements**, are not covered by insurance, making them financially inaccessible to some people. Even if they are covered, many alternative treatments require multiple sessions or long-term use of supplements, leading to high out-of-pocket costs. For individuals without insurance or those with limited financial resources, these treatments may become a financial burden, making it harder for them to access conventional medical care that could address the root causes of their health issues.

In conclusion, while alternative medicine offers a wide array of therapies with potential benefits, it also comes with risks that must be carefully considered. From the lack of scientific evidence and potential adverse reactions to the possibility of delaying necessary medical treatment and being misled by unqualified practitioners, it's important to approach alternative therapies with caution. Ensuring that any alternative treatment is used safely, under the guidance of qualified practitioners, and in conjunction with conventional medical care is crucial for minimizing risks and achieving the best possible health outcomes. As with any healthcare decision, thorough research, open communication with healthcare providers, and a balanced approach are key to safely incorporating alternative medicine into a person's wellness plan.

Ethical Issues

The use of alternative medicine raises several ethical issues that can affect both patients and healthcare providers. These concerns often revolve around **patient safety, informed consent, misleading claims**, and the **integration** of alternative therapies with conventional medicine. As interest in alternative treatments grows, it's important to address these ethical considerations to ensure that patients receive safe, effective, and transparent care.

One of the key ethical issues is **informed consent**. Patients seeking alternative treatments need to be fully informed about the potential benefits and risks of a therapy. Informed consent involves ensuring that the patient understands the nature of the treatment, any possible side effects, its scientific validity, and its potential interactions with conventional medications. In many cases, alternative therapies lack the same level of regulation and standardized dosages as conventional medicine, which can create uncertainty about their safety and efficacy. When patients are not provided with accurate information about the effectiveness of alternative therapies, it compromises their ability to make informed choices about their health. This becomes particularly important when patients choose alternative treatments instead of conventional care for serious medical conditions, like cancer or heart disease, where timely medical intervention is critical.

Another ethical concern is **misleading claims** made by some alternative medicine practitioners. Because the field is often less regulated than conventional medicine, certain practitioners may make exaggerated or unsubstantiated claims about the effectiveness of their treatments. For example, some alternative medicine providers may promise "cures" for chronic diseases, which can create unrealistic expectations and lead patients to forgo proven therapies in favor of unproven treatments. These misleading claims can lead to significant harm, as patients may delay seeking medical attention or may not receive the appropriate care for their conditions. This raises ethical questions about the responsibility of alternative medicine practitioners to provide honest and transparent information.

There is also an ethical challenge in the **integration** of alternative medicine with conventional healthcare. As integrative medicine becomes more popular, patients may seek out alternative therapies while continuing with their prescribed medications or medical treatments. While integrative approaches can be beneficial, a lack of communication between alternative and conventional practitioners can lead to **treatment conflicts** or **drug interactions** that may not be immediately apparent to the patient. For instance, certain herbs or supplements may interfere with prescribed medications, resulting in adverse effects. The ethical responsibility of both conventional and alternative healthcare providers is to collaborate and share information to ensure that the patient's safety is not compromised. This requires an openness to different treatment approaches and a commitment to the patient's well-being.

Vulnerable populations are another group at risk when it comes to alternative medicine. Individuals dealing with chronic illness, pain, or mental health conditions may be particularly susceptible to seeking alternative treatments out of desperation or dissatisfaction with conventional medicine. In these situations, vulnerable patients may be more inclined to believe in unproven therapies, especially when offered by practitioners who provide emotional support alongside their treatments. This situation raises concerns about **exploitation**. Practitioners who take advantage of a patient's vulnerability for financial gain, or who offer therapies with no proven benefit, are engaging in unethical practices. The ethical obligation is to avoid taking advantage of a patient's emotional state and to ensure that they are given treatments based on evidence and compassion.

The ethical issue of **accessibility** is also critical. Many alternative therapies, such as **acupuncture**, **chiropractic care**, or **herbal supplements**, are not typically covered by insurance, which can limit access for individuals without the financial means to afford these treatments. This can lead to **health disparities**, where wealthier individuals have greater access to alternative medicine while underserved populations may be excluded. Additionally, some alternative treatments may require ongoing care or expensive supplements, which can further burden individuals already struggling with healthcare costs. The ethical dilemma here is ensuring that all patients have equal access to a variety of treatments that could potentially improve their health outcomes, whether they are conventional or alternative.

Lastly, the **professional responsibility** of alternative medicine practitioners is a key ethical issue. Many alternative medicine practices are not subject to the same regulatory oversight as conventional healthcare. This raises questions about the qualifications and competence of some practitioners. Without appropriate training or certification, some individuals may provide treatments that are unsafe or ineffective, putting patients at risk. Ethical practice in alternative medicine requires that practitioners have the necessary education, skills, and experience to provide safe and effective treatments. Additionally, alternative medicine practitioners must adhere to ethical standards of care, including respect for patient autonomy and the confidentiality of their medical information.

In conclusion, the ethical issues surrounding alternative medicine are multifaceted, involving considerations of patient safety, informed consent, misleading claims, and the integration of alternative and conventional therapies. As the popularity of alternative treatments continues to rise, it is essential for practitioners to be transparent about the risks and benefits of their therapies, for healthcare providers to collaborate effectively, and for vulnerable patients to be protected from exploitation. These ethical principles help ensure that alternative medicine is practiced with integrity, respect for patients, and a focus on improving health outcomes.

Regulations and Guidelines

Regulations and guidelines for alternative medicine are critical to ensuring that these therapies are both safe and effective. Since alternative medicine encompasses a broad range of practices, from **herbal medicine** and **acupuncture** to **chiropractic care** and **energy healing**, the level of regulation varies widely depending on the type of treatment and the country in which it is practiced. The absence of a unified global regulatory framework for alternative medicine makes it essential to have specific guidelines and oversight to protect both patients and practitioners.

In many countries, **herbal medicine** is subject to varying degrees of regulation. In the United States, for example, herbal products are classified as **dietary supplements** rather than medicines, which means they do not undergo the same rigorous testing and approval process required for pharmaceuticals by the **Food and Drug Administration (FDA)**. While the FDA can intervene if a product is found to be unsafe or misleadingly marketed, it does not pre-approve herbal products before they hit the market. This regulatory gap means that consumers are often left to navigate the safety and efficacy of these products on their own. In contrast, countries like Germany and the United Kingdom have stricter regulations in place, requiring more substantial evidence of safety and efficacy for herbal medicines before they are allowed for sale to the public. These regulations are typically enforced by government bodies like the **European Medicines Agency (EMA)** and the **Medicines and Healthcare products Regulatory Agency (MHRA)** in the UK, which set standards for manufacturing, labeling, and clinical trials.

For practices like **acupuncture** and **chiropractic care**, regulations tend to be more defined. In many countries, acupuncture is performed by licensed practitioners who have completed rigorous training in traditional practices, often including modern medical knowledge. For example, in the United States, acupuncture is regulated at the state level, with most states requiring acupuncturists to pass national certification exams administered by the **National Certification Commission for Acupuncture and Oriental Medicine (NCCAOM)**. Similarly, in the United Kingdom, acupuncture practitioners must be registered with an accredited body like the **British Acupuncture Council** to ensure their training and practice meet national standards.

Chiropractic care is another field that is subject to specific regulations. In the United States, chiropractors are licensed by state boards and must complete a Doctor of Chiropractic (DC) program at an accredited college, followed by national board exams. In addition to licensure, chiropractors are also held to standards set by organizations like the **American Chiropractic Association (ACA)**, which provides guidelines for professional practice, ethics, and patient care. In some countries, chiropractic care is included in national health systems, reflecting a level of regulatory acceptance and integration with conventional healthcare. In contrast, other regions may have limited regulation or fewer recognized qualifications for chiropractic practitioners.

Energy healing practices, such as **Reiki** and **therapeutic touch**, are generally less regulated than more established practices like acupuncture or chiropractic care. These therapies are often provided by unlicensed practitioners who may not have specific formal training requirements. Because energy healing practices typically do not involve the use of pharmaceutical drugs or invasive procedures, many countries do not have specific laws regulating them. However, this lack of regulation can be a concern, especially when individuals are seeking treatment for serious health conditions. Some organizations, such as the **International Association of Reiki Professionals (IARP)**, provide certification programs and guidelines to help ensure that practitioners are properly trained. However, these guidelines are not legally enforced and often rely on voluntary adherence by practitioners.

In terms of **integrative medicine**, where conventional and alternative treatments are combined, healthcare practitioners must often follow the regulatory guidelines of both systems. For instance, medical doctors practicing integrative medicine may need to adhere to traditional medical standards while also integrating alternative therapies, such as acupuncture or nutritional counseling, into their practices. Many integrative medicine centers and practitioners are subject to local healthcare laws and standards, and they may also receive accreditation from professional organizations that set specific guidelines for combining alternative and conventional medicine. The **American Board of Integrative Medicine (ABIM)**, for example, certifies physicians in integrative medicine after they meet certain educational and professional criteria.

At the global level, there is no unified regulatory body for alternative medicine, and the standards for practice and training can vary widely between countries. The **World Health Organization (WHO)** has taken steps toward establishing guidelines for traditional medicine, including acupuncture and herbal medicine, but these are not legally binding. The WHO's efforts aim to ensure that traditional practices are safe, effective, and evidence-based, helping to standardize treatments and protect patients. Similarly, the **World**

Federation of Chiropractic (WFC) works to promote regulatory standards for chiropractic care across the globe, encouraging countries to adopt similar guidelines for licensing and practice.

Despite these efforts, significant challenges remain in the regulation of alternative medicine. One key challenge is the **lack of consistency** in training and certification across different modalities and countries. Without standardized education or certification, patients may have difficulty identifying qualified practitioners, leading to a lack of trust in the safety of alternative therapies. Moreover, the varying levels of regulation can lead to situations where practitioners who do not meet high professional standards continue to offer services, potentially putting patients at risk.

In conclusion, while there are increasing efforts to regulate and standardize alternative medicine practices, the lack of universal guidelines remains a significant issue. Patients seeking alternative therapies should be cautious, researching the qualifications of practitioners and ensuring that the treatments are supported by scientific evidence. Governments, professional organizations, and regulatory bodies must continue to work together to create clearer, more consistent standards for alternative medicine to protect patients and improve the integration of these therapies into the broader healthcare system.

The Future of Alternative Medicine

The future of alternative medicine appears promising, as growing interest in holistic approaches to health continues to shape both the healthcare landscape and patient expectations. As more people seek natural, non-invasive therapies to complement or even replace traditional treatments, the integration of alternative medicine into mainstream healthcare is becoming increasingly viable. However, the future of this field will depend on advancements in scientific research, regulation, and the continued collaboration between conventional and alternative practitioners.

One of the key trends in the future of alternative medicine is **increased integration with conventional healthcare**. As research continues to support the efficacy of many alternative therapies, particularly in areas like pain management, chronic disease management, and mental health, alternative medicine is likely to become a more common part of integrative care models. **Integrative medicine**, which blends conventional treatments with alternative therapies, is already gaining traction in healthcare systems worldwide. This approach not only helps patients access a wider range of treatments but also supports a more personalized approach to care. Over the next decade, we can expect more hospitals, clinics, and healthcare providers to offer integrative options, allowing patients to benefit from both conventional and alternative methods under one roof.

Scientific research will continue to play a crucial role in the evolution of alternative medicine. As demand for alternative therapies rises, so too will the need for rigorous studies to confirm the safety and efficacy of these treatments. We can anticipate further research into the benefits of **acupuncture, herbal medicine, mind-body therapies**, and other alternative practices. More clinical trials, meta-analyses, and large-scale studies will help clarify how these therapies work, who they benefit most, and how they can be safely integrated with conventional medicine. The development of standardized protocols for alternative treatments, backed by evidence-based research, will likely drive acceptance and increase the integration of alternative therapies into conventional medical settings.

In particular, the **use of technology** will have a significant impact on the future of alternative medicine. With advancements in **telemedicine** and **virtual care**, patients will have greater access to alternative therapies, such as remote consultations with **nutritionists, acupuncturists**, and **mental health professionals**. Digital platforms can provide education, virtual therapy sessions, and personalized treatment plans based on a patient's unique health needs. Moreover, the use of **artificial intelligence (AI)** in healthcare is expected to play a role in identifying the most effective alternative treatments based on individual patient data, improving the precision and customization of care. For example, AI could help analyze vast amounts of data to identify which herbal remedies are most effective for specific conditions, or which combinations of treatments work best for pain management.

Regulation and standardization of alternative medicine will be another critical area of development. As the popularity of alternative therapies increases, governments and professional organizations will likely implement stricter regulatory frameworks to ensure the safety and quality of treatments. This could involve establishing clear guidelines for training, certification, and licensing of practitioners across various alternative medicine modalities, as well as ensuring the safety and purity of herbal supplements and other products. Efforts like these would help build trust in alternative medicine, ensuring that patients have access to therapies that are both effective and safe.

With **patient-centered care** becoming the cornerstone of modern medicine, there is growing recognition of the importance of treating not just the physical body, but also emotional and mental health. Alternative medicine has long embraced this holistic approach, and as awareness of the mind-body connection continues to grow, therapies like **meditation**, **yoga**, and **acupuncture** will become increasingly integrated into mental health and wellness programs. The future may see alternative medicine expanding beyond traditional settings, such as hospitals and clinics, and becoming part of wellness programs offered in schools, workplaces, and communities. Integrating alternative therapies into mental health treatment plans could help reduce **stress**, **anxiety**, and **depression**, offering people holistic tools to maintain emotional balance in a fast-paced world.

Personalization of healthcare will also be a significant factor in the future of alternative medicine. As more research is conducted into genetic predispositions, **epigenetics**, and individual responses to different treatments, alternative medicine will likely become more tailored to the individual. Personalized treatments, based on a person's genetic makeup, lifestyle, and environmental factors, could lead to more effective therapies. For example, **nutritional counseling** and **herbal medicine** might be increasingly personalized, with treatments specifically designed to address an individual's unique biochemical makeup, ensuring better outcomes in managing chronic diseases like diabetes, heart disease, or autoimmune disorders.

Patient education and empowerment will also play a pivotal role in the future of alternative medicine. As more people seek alternatives to pharmaceutical treatments, they will become increasingly educated about the potential benefits and risks of alternative therapies. This will empower patients to make informed decisions about their care and take an active role in their health. Additionally, the rise of **online communities** and **social media** platforms has facilitated the sharing of experiences and information about alternative therapies, helping to create a more informed and connected patient base.

In summary, the future of alternative medicine is bright, characterized by greater integration with conventional healthcare, increased scientific validation, improved regulation, and a growing emphasis on personalized, patient-centered care. With advancements in technology, research, and public education, alternative medicine will continue to evolve, offering patients a broader range of options to address their health concerns. The ongoing collaboration between conventional and alternative healthcare providers promises to create a more holistic, accessible, and effective healthcare system, helping to meet the diverse needs of patients worldwide.

Emerging Trends

The field of alternative medicine is continuously evolving, with new trends and innovations emerging as more individuals seek natural, holistic approaches to health and wellness. These emerging trends reflect both advancements in scientific understanding and shifts in patient preferences, focusing on integrating alternative therapies with conventional care, enhancing accessibility, and offering personalized treatments. Here are some key trends shaping the future of alternative medicine.

One of the most significant trends is the increasing **integration of alternative medicine with conventional healthcare**. As more studies show the benefits of alternative therapies like **acupuncture, herbal medicine, mind-body practices**, and **chiropractic care**, many healthcare systems are embracing integrative medicine as a way to offer patients a more holistic approach. In integrative medicine, conventional treatments, such as prescription medications and surgery, are used alongside alternative therapies to treat the whole person—body, mind, and spirit. This trend is driven by patients seeking more options for managing chronic conditions, improving quality of life, and reducing side effects from conventional treatments. Hospitals, clinics, and wellness centers are increasingly offering a range of complementary therapies alongside traditional medical care, reflecting a growing recognition of the benefits of combining both approaches.

Another emerging trend is the rise of **personalized alternative therapies**. Advances in **genetics, epigenetics,** and **biotechnology** are enabling more individualized approaches to health and wellness. Alternative treatments, such as **nutritional counseling, herbal remedies,** and **supplementation**, are becoming more customized based on a person's unique genetic makeup, health history, and lifestyle. This trend is aligned with the broader movement toward **precision medicine**, where treatments are tailored to the individual rather than using a one-size-fits-all approach. For instance, genetic testing could help determine which herbs or supplements are most effective for a person's specific health needs, improving the efficacy of alternative treatments and reducing the risk of adverse effects.

Technology is also playing an increasingly significant role in the evolution of alternative medicine. The rise of **telemedicine** has made it easier for patients to access alternative therapies remotely, especially in areas such as **nutrition counseling, stress management, mental health therapies,** and **herbal consultations**. Through virtual consultations, individuals can receive personalized treatment plans from qualified practitioners without the need for in-person visits. Additionally, **digital health tools** like apps for **meditation, yoga,** and **biofeedback** are becoming more popular, allowing individuals to monitor their well-being and track their progress with alternative therapies. The use of **wearable devices** that measure things like **heart rate variability** and **sleep patterns** also supports the growing trend of **self-care** and **preventive health**, helping individuals take a more active role in managing their health with alternative approaches.

Mind-body practices, including **yoga, meditation,** and **mindfulness**, are becoming increasingly mainstream, particularly as awareness of mental health's impact on overall wellness grows. Studies have consistently shown the effectiveness of these therapies in reducing **stress**, improving

mental clarity, enhancing **emotional resilience**, and alleviating **chronic pain**. With a growing body of research supporting their benefits, more people are incorporating mind-body techniques into their daily routines. These practices are particularly beneficial in managing conditions like **anxiety, depression, PTSD,** and **insomnia**, and they are being integrated into both clinical and wellness settings. Mind-body practices are not only seen as effective for addressing mental health, but also for enhancing physical health, making them an integral part of modern alternative medicine.

In the realm of **herbal medicine**, there is a growing focus on **standardization** and **evidence-based practice**. As herbal remedies gain popularity, there is an increasing push for standardized dosages, quality control, and clinical validation to ensure both safety and efficacy. Regulatory bodies in some countries are implementing stricter guidelines to monitor the quality of herbal products, and research into specific herbs is expanding. For example, **turmeric, ginger,** and **ashwagandha** are being studied for their potential anti-inflammatory, antioxidant, and adaptogenic properties. More clinical trials are focusing on the use of herbs in treating chronic conditions, such as **arthritis, diabetes,** and **cancer,** and herbal treatments are often being used as complementary options alongside conventional therapies.

Functional medicine is another rapidly growing trend in alternative medicine. This patient-centered approach focuses on identifying and addressing the root causes of illness, rather than simply managing symptoms. Functional medicine practitioners often use **dietary changes, nutritional supplements, lifestyle adjustments,** and **detoxification protocols** to treat chronic conditions such as **autoimmune diseases, gastrointestinal disorders,** and **hormonal imbalances**. This holistic approach considers the interaction between genetics, environment, and lifestyle in the development of disease, and is increasingly popular among patients who are seeking more individualized care. Functional medicine is gaining acceptance not only in alternative medicine circles but also among mainstream healthcare providers who recognize the importance of treating the whole person.

In addition, there is growing interest in **integrating alternative medicine into mental health care**. As mental health issues like **anxiety**, **depression**, and **stress** continue to rise, many individuals are turning to alternative treatments to complement or supplement traditional therapies. **Acupuncture, aromatherapy, Reiki**, and **herbal supplements** are being used alongside psychotherapy and medications to help manage symptoms and improve emotional well-being. Mindfulness-based therapies and **cognitive behavioral therapy (CBT)**, which have their roots in alternative practices, are now being widely recognized and integrated into mainstream mental health care as effective tools for reducing anxiety and improving mood regulation.

Finally, the increasing demand for **sustainability** is influencing alternative medicine trends. As more individuals become conscious of the environmental impact of pharmaceuticals, there is growing interest in natural remedies that are both effective and environmentally friendly. **Eco-conscious** herbal medicine practices, sustainable **acupuncture needle disposal**, and **green wellness centers** are emerging trends in response to this demand. Consumers are becoming more aware of the sourcing and environmental footprint of the products they use, prompting companies to adopt more sustainable practices in the production of alternative medicine products and treatments.

In conclusion, emerging trends in alternative medicine are characterized by increased integration with conventional care, advances in personalized treatments, the use of technology to enhance accessibility, and a growing emphasis on mind-body practices. As scientific research continues to validate the effectiveness of many alternative therapies, and as the public continues to seek holistic, personalized approaches to health, alternative medicine will play an increasingly important role in healthcare. The future of alternative medicine will be shaped by these trends, ultimately making natural, integrative treatments more accessible, effective, and accepted in mainstream healthcare.

Impact on Healthcare System

The rise of alternative medicine has had a notable impact on the healthcare system, influencing everything from patient care and treatment options to the way healthcare professionals approach wellness. As more individuals seek non-invasive, natural therapies alongside or in place of conventional treatments, alternative medicine is reshaping the landscape of modern healthcare. This shift is not without challenges, but it has prompted important changes that are enhancing the overall approach to patient care, improving access to diverse treatment options, and fostering a more integrative model of healthcare.

One significant impact of alternative medicine on the healthcare system is the **increased demand for integrative medicine**. As patients look for more holistic approaches to their health, many healthcare systems are incorporating alternative therapies alongside conventional treatments to create a more comprehensive model of care. **Integrative medicine** combines treatments like **acupuncture, herbal medicine, chiropractic care**, and **mind-body therapies** with standard medical practices such as pharmaceuticals and surgery. This approach has gained traction in hospitals, wellness centers, and private practices, as more patients demand alternatives to traditional medications, particularly for chronic conditions, pain management, and mental health issues. Integrative clinics and departments are becoming increasingly common, reflecting the growing trend to treat the whole person, not just the symptoms.

This shift toward integrative care has also led to **greater collaboration** between conventional medical professionals and alternative medicine practitioners. As more research supports the benefits of treatments like acupuncture and herbal remedies, there is growing recognition that these therapies can complement traditional medical care. Healthcare providers are beginning to work together with alternative medicine practitioners to provide well-rounded care for patients, offering a broader array of treatment options. For example, a patient undergoing chemotherapy might receive **acupuncture** to help alleviate nausea or **nutrition counseling** to support their immune system. This integration fosters a more patient-centered approach and emphasizes the importance of treating both the body and mind.

Alternative medicine has also led to **improvements in patient empowerment and involvement** in healthcare decisions. With increasing access to information about alternative therapies, many patients are taking a more active role in their health. This trend is particularly evident in the management of **chronic diseases**, where patients are seeking alternative therapies to complement conventional treatments. For instance, individuals with **arthritis** may use **herbal supplements** and **physical therapies** like **yoga** to manage symptoms, while those with **chronic pain** might turn to **acupuncture** or **chiropractic care**. As patients become more involved in their treatment choices, healthcare providers are learning to adapt by offering more personalized and flexible care plans that include both conventional and alternative options.

Another important change in the healthcare system due to alternative medicine is its **potential to reduce healthcare costs**. Many alternative therapies, such as **acupuncture**,

chiropractic care, and **massage therapy**, focus on **prevention**, **wellness**, and the management of chronic conditions rather than the treatment of acute symptoms. By addressing issues like pain, stress, and inflammation early, these therapies may reduce the need for expensive interventions such as surgery or long-term medications. For example, chiropractic care for back pain or acupuncture for migraines can reduce reliance on painkillers, which can be costly and come with significant side effects. As the focus shifts more toward prevention and holistic care, the overall cost burden on the healthcare system may decrease, especially as more people embrace **self-care** and **preventive health** practices.

Despite these benefits, the impact of alternative medicine on the healthcare system also raises several challenges. One major challenge is the **lack of regulation** and standardization in many alternative practices. While some forms of alternative medicine, like acupuncture and chiropractic care, are regulated and require professional training and licensure, other therapies, such as **Reiki** or **herbal supplements**, are often unregulated. This inconsistency can make it difficult for patients to know which practitioners are qualified and which treatments are safe. Furthermore, the **lack of scientific evidence** for certain alternative therapies can make it difficult to integrate them into evidence-based medical practices. This gap in research means that healthcare providers may be hesitant to recommend alternative treatments without concrete evidence of their safety and efficacy.

There are also concerns about **patient safety** when alternative therapies are used alongside conventional treatments. Some herbal remedies, for example, can interact with prescription medications, leading to potential complications. **St. John's Wort**, often used for depression, can interfere with the effectiveness of antidepressants, birth control, and blood thinners. Similarly, certain herbs may exacerbate health problems or interfere with standard treatments for chronic conditions like diabetes or high blood pressure. These potential risks highlight the need for better collaboration and communication between conventional medical providers and alternative practitioners to ensure that patients are not unknowingly putting their health at risk.

Finally, the **cost of alternative treatments** can be a barrier to widespread adoption, especially when these therapies are not covered by insurance. Many patients seeking alternative therapies may face financial challenges, particularly if they require ongoing treatments, such as acupuncture or chiropractic care. While alternative medicine can often be more affordable than conventional treatments in some areas, its lack of insurance coverage makes it less accessible for those without the financial means to pay out-of-pocket for these services.

In conclusion, the rise of alternative medicine has had a profound impact on the healthcare system, fostering greater collaboration, improving patient empowerment, and encouraging more holistic approaches to health. By integrating alternative therapies with conventional care, the healthcare system is becoming more patient-centered and diverse in the treatment options it provides. However, challenges remain, including the need for better regulation, standardization, and evidence to support alternative therapies. As the field continues to evolve, the healthcare system will need to adapt to ensure that alternative medicine can be safely and effectively integrated into broader health strategies, ultimately enhancing the quality of care and improving outcomes for patients.

Personalized Alternative Treatment

Personalized alternative treatment is an evolving approach that tailors therapies to the individual's unique health needs, preferences, and genetic makeup. Rather than offering a one-size-fits-all solution, this method considers the specific characteristics of the person, including their lifestyle, medical history, and even genetic predispositions, to create a more effective and customized healing plan. This personalized approach is gaining traction within the alternative medicine community, offering a more holistic and targeted path to wellness.

One of the key aspects of personalized alternative treatment is the use of **genetic testing** and **biomarker analysis**. By analyzing an individual's genetic makeup, practitioners can determine how a person is likely to respond to certain treatments, whether they be **herbal remedies**, **nutritional plans**, or **acupuncture**. For instance, some people may metabolize certain herbs or medications more efficiently due to their genetic profile, while others may be more sensitive to specific compounds. Personalized herbal medicine takes into account these genetic factors to optimize the use of plants and natural remedies that are most likely to benefit the patient. This approach ensures that the remedies chosen are both effective and safe, minimizing the risk of adverse effects.

In addition to genetic factors, **lifestyle and environmental factors** are integral to personalized alternative treatments. These factors include diet, physical activity, stress levels, sleep habits, and exposure to environmental toxins. For example, an individual with **chronic fatigue** may benefit from a combination of **nutritional supplements** like **B vitamins** and **adaptogenic herbs** like **ashwagandha** to support energy levels. At the same time, lifestyle modifications, such as implementing a regular **sleep routine** or reducing **stress** through **mindfulness meditation**, may be incorporated into the treatment plan. Personalized treatment recognizes that improving overall well-being involves addressing all aspects of an individual's life.

Personalized treatments also take into account the unique **mind-body connection**. Many alternative medicine practices, such as **yoga**, **meditation**, and **Reiki**, focus on balancing the emotional and psychological aspects of health. For individuals experiencing **anxiety**, **depression**, or **stress-related illnesses**, a personalized treatment plan may incorporate **cognitive-behavioral therapy (CBT)** alongside practices like **mindfulness-based stress reduction (MBSR)** or **breathing exercises**. These therapies are tailored to fit the emotional and mental needs of the patient, helping them manage stress more effectively and achieve a balanced state of mind.

The role of **nutrition** in personalized alternative medicine is another critical component. A diet that aligns with an individual's genetic makeup and health needs can be a powerful tool in managing chronic conditions, preventing disease, and improving overall health. **Personalized nutrition** uses genetic testing, metabolic data, and an individual's specific health conditions to design meal plans and supplement regimens that support optimal wellness. For instance, someone with a **genetic predisposition to high cholesterol** might benefit from a diet high in **omega-3 fatty acids** and **fiber-rich**

foods to support heart health. Similarly, those with digestive issues may be prescribed a **low FODMAP diet** or **probiotic supplements** based on their unique gut microbiome and digestive health.

Another area where personalized alternative treatment is making strides is in **chronic pain management**. Traditional approaches to pain management often rely on generic medications or procedures that may not address the root cause of the problem. Personalized pain management in alternative medicine takes a more targeted approach, integrating therapies like **acupuncture, chiropractic care, massage**, and **herbal remedies** tailored to the individual's condition. For example, someone suffering from **musculoskeletal pain** may benefit from **acupuncture** to target specific points of discomfort, combined with **anti-inflammatory herbs** like **turmeric** and **ginger** to reduce swelling. Additionally, personalized **movement therapies**, such as tailored **yoga poses** or physical therapy exercises, can help restore mobility and alleviate pain.

Epigenetics, the study of how lifestyle and environmental factors influence gene expression, is an emerging field that complements personalized alternative treatments. Epigenetic factors play a role in how the body responds to stress, diet, exercise, and even toxins. Personalized alternative treatments that incorporate epigenetic insights may offer new ways to address conditions like **autoimmune diseases, cardiovascular disease**, and **chronic inflammation**. By understanding how environmental factors influence gene expression, practitioners can recommend specific lifestyle changes, herbs, and dietary adjustments to help support optimal gene expression and reduce disease risk.

Another innovation in personalized alternative treatments is the use of **holistic health assessments** that consider the whole person. Practitioners may use a combination of **traditional**

diagnostic methods, such as pulse diagnosis and tongue inspection (common in **Traditional Chinese Medicine**), alongside modern diagnostic tools like **blood tests**, **gut microbiome analysis**, and **hormone level assessments**. These assessments allow practitioners to gain a more comprehensive understanding of a patient's health, leading to more precise and individualized treatment plans.

Personalized alternative medicine is also becoming more **accessible** thanks to technological advancements. Virtual consultations with **holistic health practitioners**, online courses for **meditation** or **yoga**, and telemedicine platforms for personalized **nutritional guidance** are making it easier for people to access tailored treatments from the comfort of their own homes. These digital tools are helping to break down barriers to alternative care, allowing patients to receive individualized support no matter where they live.

In conclusion, personalized alternative treatment offers a promising future for healthcare by recognizing and addressing the unique needs of each individual. By incorporating genetic, lifestyle, emotional, and environmental factors into a customized treatment plan, this approach has the potential to improve outcomes, enhance patient satisfaction, and provide more effective solutions for managing chronic conditions and promoting overall wellness. As research continues to validate the effectiveness of personalized alternative therapies, and as technology makes these treatments more accessible, this model of care will likely play an increasingly important role in the healthcare system.

Have Questions / Comments?

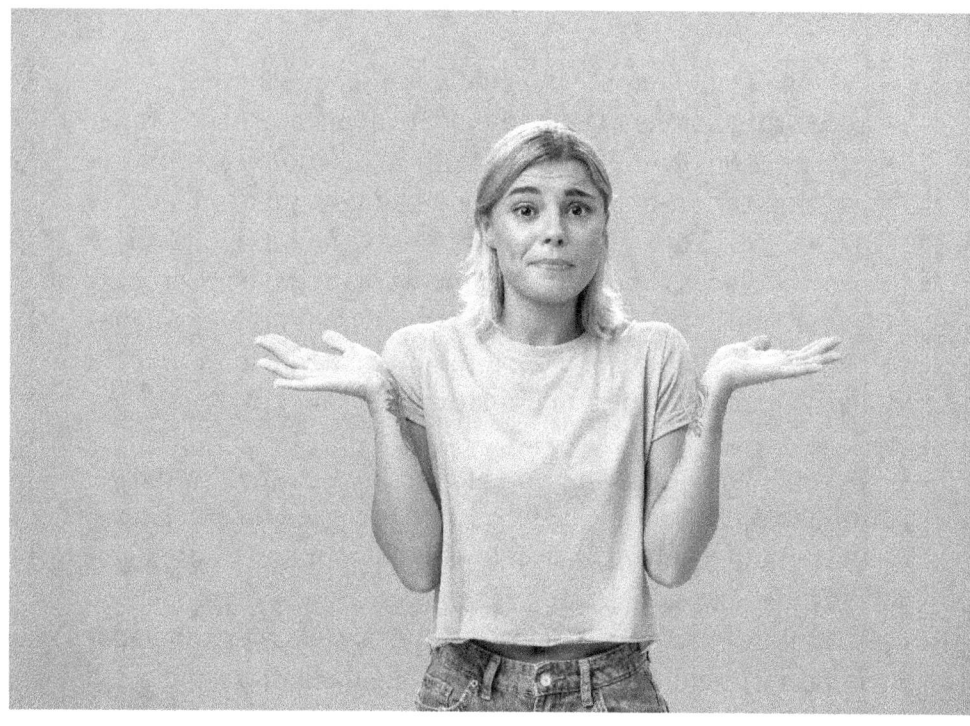

This book was designed to cover as much as possible but I know I have probably missed something, or some new amazing discovery that has just come out.

If you notice something missing or have a question that I failed to answer, please get in touch and let me know. If I can, I will email you an answer and also update the book so others can also benefit from it.

Thanks For Being Awesome :)

Submit Your Questions / Comments At:

https://questions.xspurts.com

Get Another Book Free

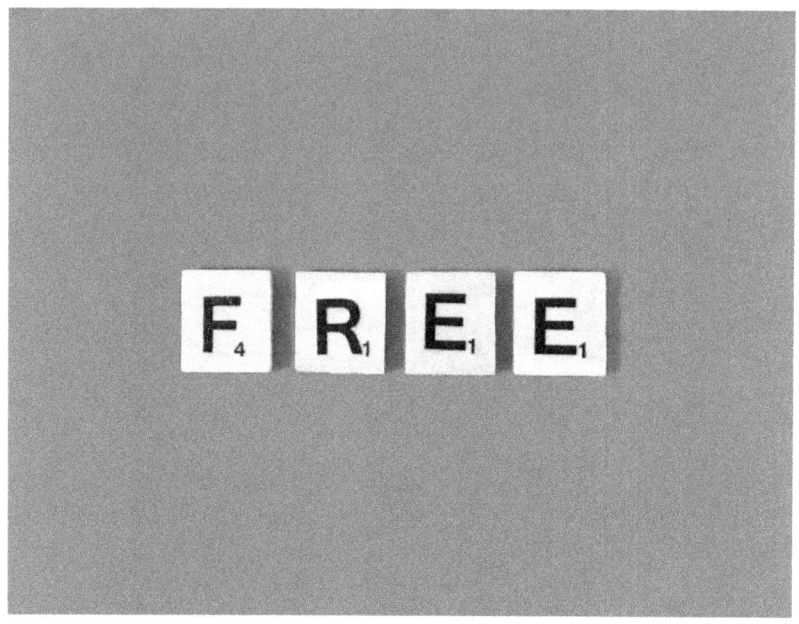

We love writing and have produced a huge number of books.

For being one of our amazing readers, we would love to offer you another book we have created, 100% free.

To claim this limited time special offer, simply go to the site below and enter your name and email address.

You will then receive one of my great books, direct to your email account, 100% free!

https://free.xspurts.com

www.ingramcontent.com/pod-product-compliance
Lightning Source LLC
Chambersburg PA
CBHW052146220526
45471CB00004B/1541